THE HAIRY *Dieters*

FAST & FRESH

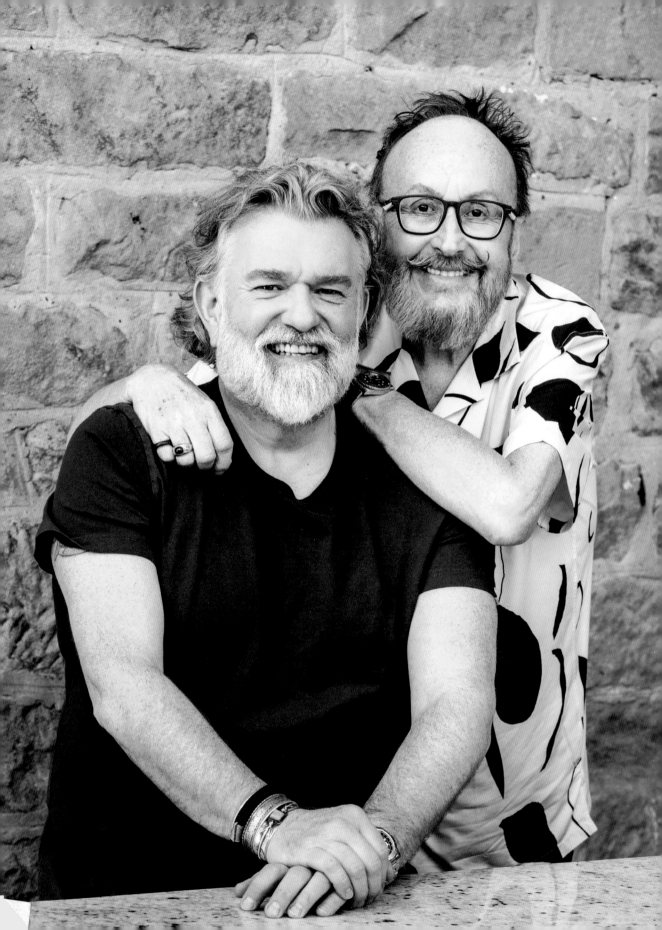

SI KING & DAVE MYERS

THE HAIRY *Dieters*

FAST &
FRESH

CONT

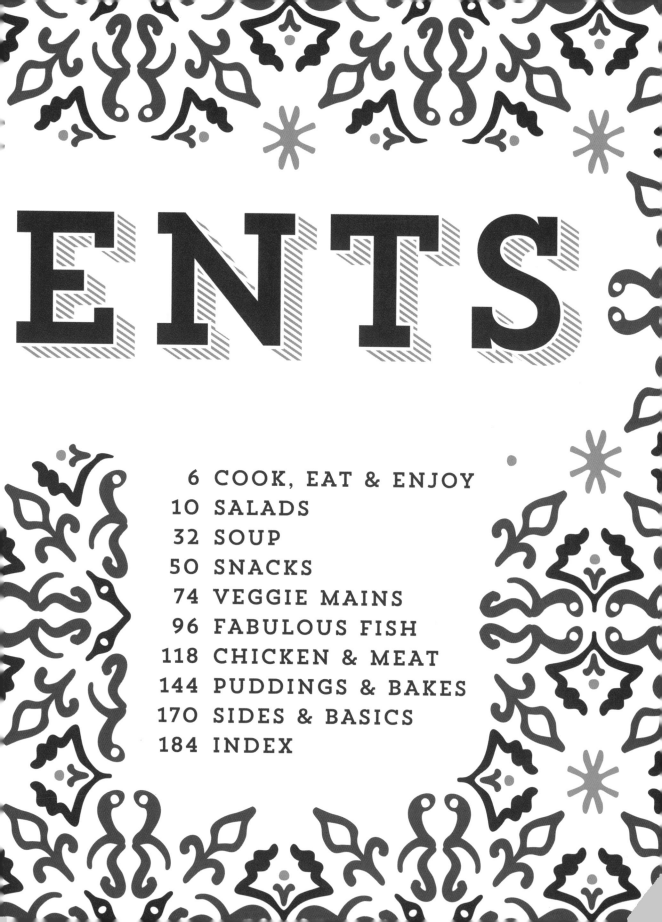

ENTS

COOK, EAT & ENJOY!

Since we wrote our first 'Hairy Dieters' book, twelve years ago, we've done our best to stay in control of our weight and our health while still enjoying great food. OK, we continue to love our pies, our cakes and a full English occasionally, but we focus on keeping to the 80:20 rule – making sure that 80 per cent of what we eat is healthy.

The easiest route to healthy eating is to cook most of our meals from scratch, using good fresh ingredients. That way you really can't go wrong. Cooking from scratch doesn't have to take lots of time and effort. There are plenty of meals in this book that can be put together in half an hour or so and reward you with bags of great flavour. Dishes such as pasta with chilli and lentils, Mediterranean chicken stir-fry, loads of quick and tasty soups, salads and snacks and even a few reasonably guilt-free sweet treats.

One of our main sources of inspiration for this book has been all the information you hear about the huge benefits of following the Mediterranean way of eating. Over and over again, scientific research shows that the Mediterranean diet is the way to a long and healthy life. It's said to reduce the risk of heart attacks, strokes, diabetes and many other conditions and to improve overall health. In various studies it has also proved to be a diet people find it easier to stick to than other regimes, such as low-fat and low-carb diets.

But don't think that eating the Mediterranean way means stuffing yourself with lots of pizza, lasagne and moussaka. That's not the answer. Key factors are focusing on eating plenty of vegetables, beans and lentils, fruit, nuts and whole grains as well as seafood, small amounts of meat and chicken and some dairy, such as cheese and plain yoghurt. Another essential is olive oil, preferably extra virgin olive oil.

Experts have identified certain areas of the world – not all in the Mediterranean but sharing a similar diet and way of life – where an unusually high number of people live to 100 and beyond. The recipes in this book are not all classic Med dishes but they use the same principles and are rich in fresh vegetables, pulses and whole grains. They are inspired by food from all over the Middle East, North Africa and even Asia and Mexico, as well as Italy, Greece, France and Spain. That doesn't mean it's all about aubergines and red peppers – traditional British favourite veggies like leeks, carrots, cabbage and cauliflower are just as good for us and delicious to eat.

As always, we've made these recipes as simple and straightforward as possible. Most don't take long to prepare – although a few do need a bit of time in the oven or to marinate – but then we believe that making dinner shouldn't always be a race against time. This is not an ultra-low-cal book as such, but we have reduced the amount of butter, sugar and other high-calorie ingredients as far as possible without compromising on flavour. And many of the dishes are under 500 calories per serving.

An important thing to bear in mind is that research has also revealed that the success of the Mediterranean diet for good health is not only down to the food. It's also about having an active lifestyle, cooking your own food and enjoying meals together round the table. Food is not just fuel, it should be a pleasure, an important part of your day, so take the chance to relax and really savour a meal as often as you can. And we're well up for that – hope you'll join us!

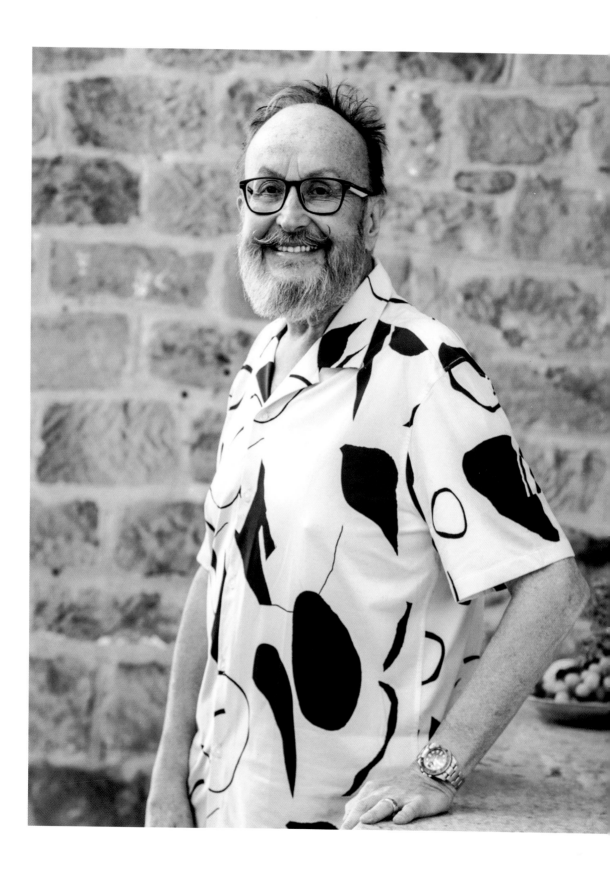

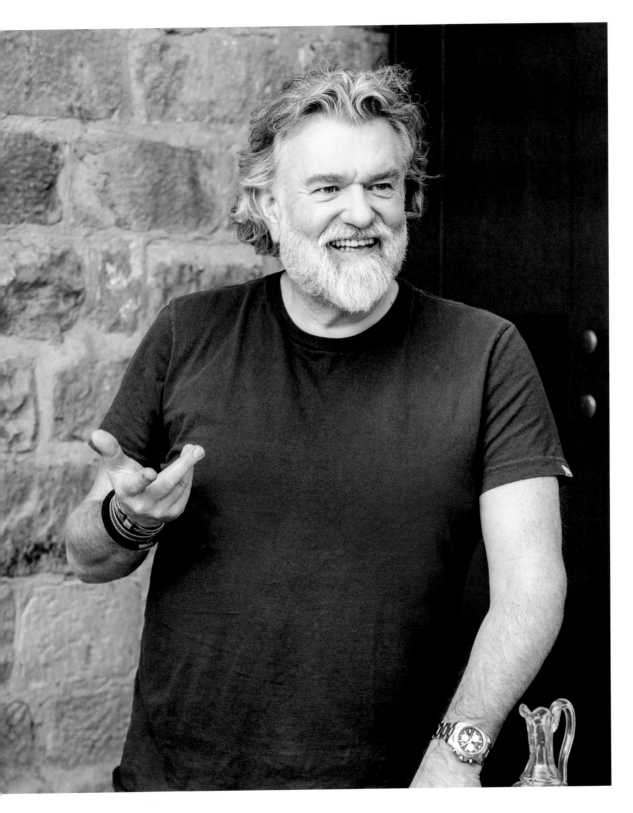

NUTRITIONAL INFO

Full nutritional info is given for each recipe in the book. Unless otherwise noted, the figures are per serving, without any optional extras.

- **Calories** measure the amount of energy in the food. It can be tedious and not necessary to count calories every day, but it's useful to know the dangerous calorie-bomb foods. Everyone should know the approximate number of calories in the food they eat.

- **Protein** helps you feel satisfied, and we need protein to maintain our body's processes. Nuts and pulses, as well as meat, fish, eggs and dairy, are all good sources.

- **Carbohydrates** are made up of lots of sugar molecules bound together. Your digestion will turn them into sugar. But some are digested faster than others – and slowly digested carbs, like wholegrain foods, are easier for your body to handle. The huge problem is added sugar in highly processed foods, such as ready meals and takeaways. By avoiding processed foods, you'll benefit more than by worrying about different types of carbs.

- **Sugar** – figures listed are for the total sugar in a dish, which includes the natural sugars in fruit, vegetables and dairy. It is the added sugar or free sugar, like the sugar added to tea or used in puddings, that we need to limit for weight loss and good health.

- **Fat** – this figure is the total fat contained in a serving (monounsaturated, polyunsaturated and saturated).

Monounsaturated fat – in foods such as nuts, seeds and olive oil – and polyunsaturated fats in oily fish are better for you than saturated fat but they are still high in calories. Fats are made up of strings of carbon atoms with lots of energy stored in the links between them. Gram for gram they are the most calorie-dense food.

- **Saturated fats** have different links between the carbon atoms (they are 'saturated' with hydrogen atoms). They are less healthy inside the body, but most people – even experts – don't realise that any excess carbohydrate is turned into 100 per cent saturated fat in the body, whereas butter is only around 50 per cent saturated fat. The total amount of food eaten matters more than the type of fat in food.

- **Fibre** is not digested and so does not add calories. It is contained in plant foods, such as fruit, vegetables, nuts and seeds, as well as in grains and we need a good amount of fibre in the diet to help digestion. Wholegrain bread, brown rice and brown pasta contain more fibre than refined varieties.

- **Salt** – the figures given are for the salt content in the ingredients, not any extra added to taste.

A FEW NOTES FROM US

- Follow the recipes carefully so you don't change the calorie count or nutritional details. Weigh your ingredients and use measuring spoons and a measuring jug.

- Use free-range eggs whenever possible. We generally use large eggs unless otherwise specified.

- We've made oven temperatures as accurate as possible, but all ovens are different, so keep an eye on your dish and cook it for a longer or shorter time if necessary.

- Peel vegetables, onions and garlic unless otherwise specified in the recipe.

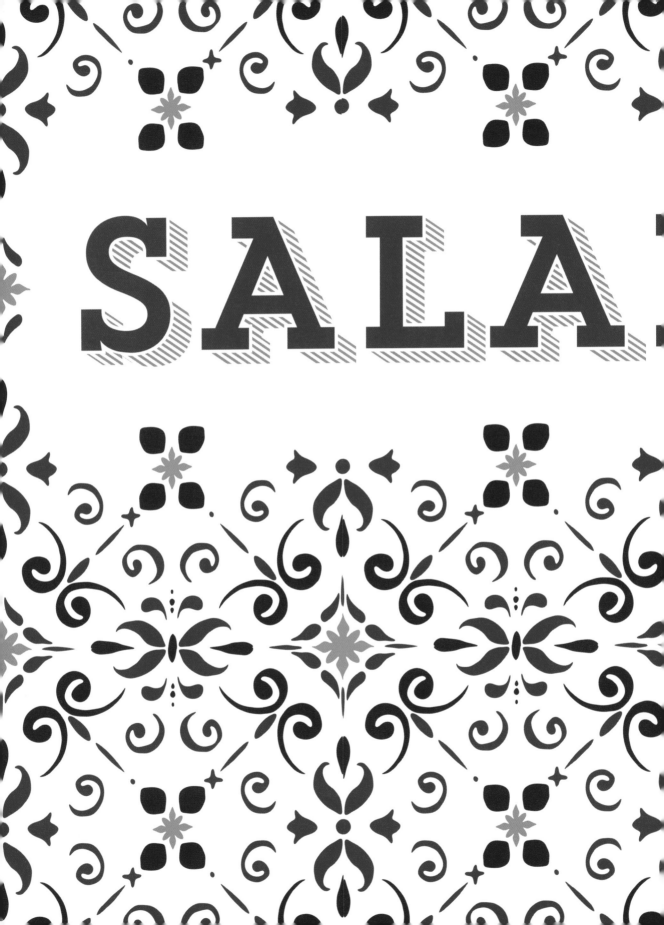

AUTUMN PANZANELLA

RED PEPPER SALAD WITH FETA

BEAN & BULGUR WHEAT SALAD

CAULIFLOWER, BROCCOLI & COUSCOUS SALAD

ROAST CARROT & RED CABBAGE SALAD

PUTTANESCA-STYLE PASTA SALAD

WHITE BEAN & TUNA SALAD

SQUID, PRAWN & BLACK BEAN SALAD

CHICKEN & FREEKEH SALAD

GRILLED BEEF & BEETROOT SALAD

Serves: **4**

 Prep: **15 minutes, plus standing time**

 Cooking time: **about 35 minutes**

 Calories per serving: **430**

AUTUMN PANZANELLA

ROAST VEGETABLES

500g squash

2 red onions, cut into wedges

a few garlic cloves

1 tsp dried thyme

½ tsp chilli flakes

1 tbsp olive oil

SALAD

200g tomatoes, roughly chopped

1 tbsp olive oil

250g stale sourdough or ciabatta, cubed

2 garlic cloves, finely chopped

100g salad leaves

50g black pitted olives

25g pumpkin seeds, lightly toasted

salt and black pepper

DRESSING

2 tbsp olive oil

1 tbsp apple balsamic or sherry vinegar

We've always been very fond of a classic panzanella salad in the summer, so we wanted to come up with a more autumnal version. We decided to add some nice roasted squash and onions to the tomatoes, leaves and olives for a more robust dish. No need to take the peel off the squash before roasting and it's up to you whether you remove it before serving. It does provide a bit of extra fibre.

Preheat the oven to 200°C/Fan 180°C/Gas 6. Wash and dry the squash, then cut it in half. Scoop out the seeds and membrane and discard them. Cut the flesh into wedges – no need to peel. Arrange the squash in a roasting tin with the red onions and garlic cloves, then sprinkle over the thyme and chilli flakes and drizzle with olive oil. Roast the veg in the oven for about half an hour until tender.

Meanwhile, put the tomatoes in a colander and sprinkle them with salt, then leave them to stand for half an hour. Heat the olive oil in a frying pan and add the cubes of bread. Stir-fry until they're crisp, then add the garlic and cook for another couple of minutes. Remove the pan from the heat and set the bread aside to cool down.

Put the bread in a bowl with the tomatoes and toss gently to combine. Roughly cut up the squash – removing the peel if you want – and add it to the bowl with the onions.

For the dresssing, squeeze out the flesh from the roasted garlic cloves and mix with the olive oil and vinegar. Add this to the contents of the bowl, then season with a little salt and plenty of black pepper.

Leave the salad to stand for 10 minutes, then add the salad leaves just before serving. Toss everything briefly and sprinkle over the olives and pumpkin seeds.

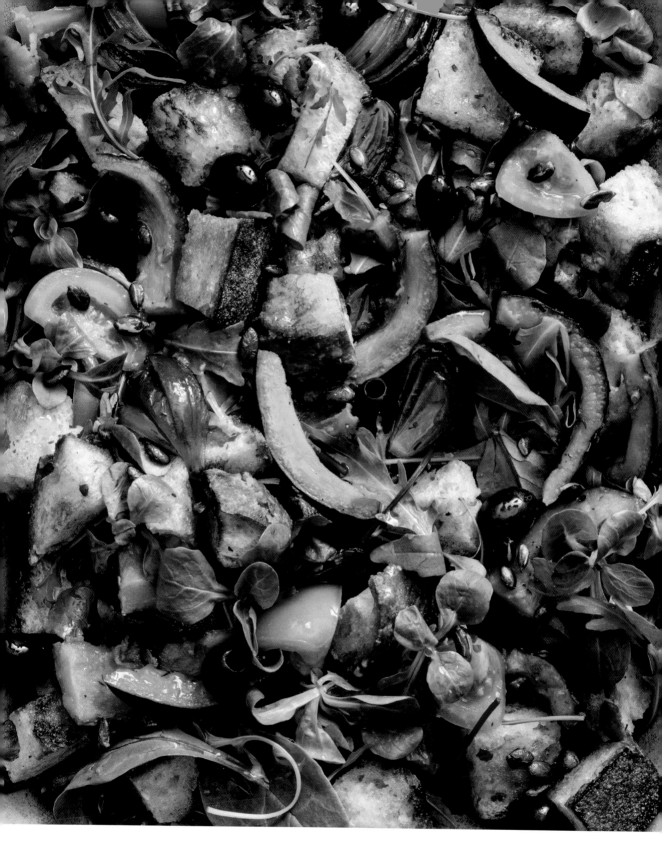

INFO PER SERVING: PROTEIN (G) 11   CARBS (G) 50.5   SUGAR (G) 14   FAT (G) 19   SATURATED FAT (G) 2.5   FIBRE (G) 8   SALT (G) 1

Serves: **4**

 Prep: **10 minutes**

 Cooking time:
about 10 minutes

 Calories per serving:
270

RED PEPPER SALAD WITH FETA

2 tbsp olive oil

3 red peppers, cut into strips

2 small red onions, cut into slim
    wedges

1 tsp dried oregano, thyme or
    mixed herbs

2 garlic cloves, finely sliced

zest of 1 lemon

150g salad leaves, such as
    rocket, baby spinach.

100g cherry tomatoes, halved

2 tbsp capers, rinsed

mint and parsley sprigs

2 tbsp pine nuts or flaked
    almonds, lightly toasted

salt and black pepper

FETA DRESSING

100g feta

1 garlic clove, crushed

50g Greek yoghurt or kefir

1 tbsp olive oil

juice of ½ lemon

1 tsp sherry vinegar

Peppers are low in calories but they're stuffed full of vitamins, particularly vitamin C, so they're really good for you as well as delicious. This colourful salad (a version of the Italian red pepper dish peperonata) is made extra special by the feta dressing and is ideal for a light lunch or to serve as one of a selection of salads for a party.

Heat the olive oil in a large sauté pan and add the red peppers and onions. Cook over a high heat for a few minutes until they are starting to soften, stirring just once or twice so they have time to take on some colour. Season with salt and pepper and sprinkle over the dried herbs, garlic and lemon zest. Cover the pan and cook over a low heat for just a few more minutes until the vegetables have softened but haven't collapsed – the core of the onions should be tender to the point of a knife. Remove the pan from the heat and leave to cool to room temperature.

For the feta dressing, crumble the feta into a small food processor and add the garlic. Process until well broken down, then add the yoghurt or kefir and blitz until smooth. Drizzle in the olive oil, lemon juice and sherry vinegar while the motor is still running. Taste and add salt and pepper if necessary.

To assemble, arrange the salad leaves in 4 bowls. Top with the peppers and onions, followed by the cherry tomatoes. Drizzle over the dressing, then top with the capers, herbs and the pine nuts or flaked almonds.

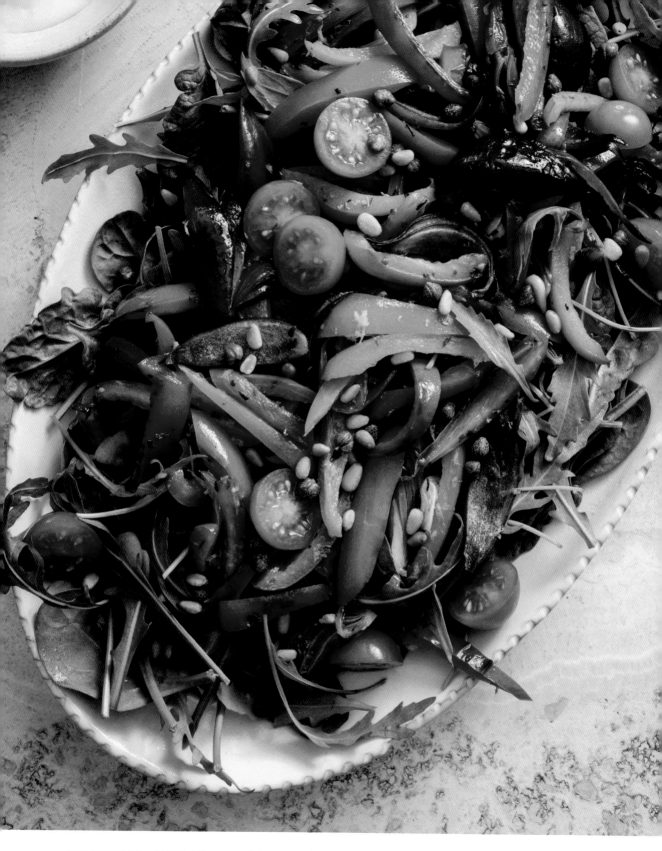

INFO PER SERVING: PROTEIN (G) 8   CARBS (G) 11   SUGAR (G) 10   FAT (G) 20   SATURATED FAT (G) 6   FIBRE (G) 5   SALT (G) 0.8

Serves: **4**

 Prep: **15 minutes, plus standing time**

 Cooking time: **about 5 minutes**

 Calories per serving with feta/without: **349/224**

BEAN & BULGUR WHEAT SALAD

50g fine bulgur wheat, well washed

100g green beans

2 x 400g cans of flageolet beans, drained and well rinsed

½ cucumber, deseeded and diced (unpeeled)

200g tomatoes, deseeded and diced

100g radishes, sliced

4 spring onions, finely sliced into rounds

small bunch of parsley, very finely chopped

small bunch of mint, leaves only, very finely chopped

200g feta (optional)

DRESSING
3 tbsp olive oil

1 tbsp red wine vinegar

zest and juice of ½ lemon

½ tsp sweet paprika

¼ tsp ground cinnamon

salt and black pepper

Bulgur wheat is very popular in Mediterranean and Middle Eastern countries and has a nice nutty flavour which pairs well with the beans in this salad. Plenty of good fibre in this one as well as lots of veg and some protein from the beans. Nice as it is or with the addition of feta to make a more substantial meal.

Cover the bulgur wheat with cold water and leave it to stand for 15 minutes, then drain thoroughly. Bring a pan of water to the boil, add the green beans and cook them for a few minutes. Drain and run the beans under cold water to stop the cooking process, then cut them into 2cm lengths.

Put the bulgur in a bowl with the green beans, flageolet beans and all the remaining vegetables. Whisk the dressing ingredients together and season with salt and pepper. Pour the dressing over the contents of the bowl, then stir in most of the herbs. Crumble over the feta, if using, then finish with the remaining herbs.

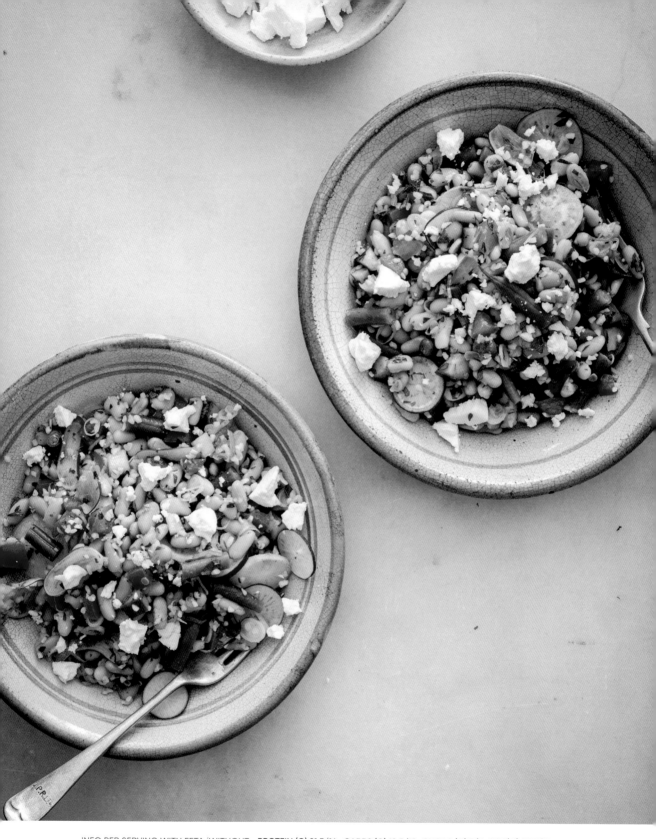

INFO PER SERVING WITH FETA/WITHOUT: PROTEIN (G) 21.5/14   CARBS (G) 18.5/18   SUGAR (G) 5/4   FAT (G) 20.5/10

SATURATED FAT (G) 8.5/1.5   FIBRE (G) 3/3   SALT (G) 1.3/0.1

Serves: **4**

 Prep: **20 minutes**

 Cooking time:
about 15 minutes

 Calories per serving:
428

COUSCOUS

50g wholegrain couscous

75ml warm water

1 tbsp olive oil

1 orange

salt and black pepper

CAULIFLOWER &
BROCCOLI

½ cauliflower, broken into small
florets

1 head of broccoli, broken into
small florets

2 tbsp olive oil

400g can of chickpeas,
drained

2 tsp baharat spice

2 garlic cloves, finely chopped

DRESSING

2 tbsp olive oil

1 tbsp sherry vinegar

zest and juice of ½ lemon

TO ASSEMBLE

100g baby spinach

1 red onion, finely sliced,
soaked in cold salted water

50g raisins, soaked in warm
water

small bunch of parsley or mint
(or both)

25g flaked almonds, lightly
toasted

1 tsp sumac

CAULIFLOWER, BROCCOLI & COUSCOUS SALAD

We find that blanching the cauli and broccoli, then sautéing them in a frying pan works well. It's a quicker method than roasting and doesn't dry the veg out. With the chickpeas and couscous, this is a really hearty salad – ideal for your lunch box.

Put the couscous in a bowl and cover it with the warm water. Season with salt and black pepper, drizzle with the oil, then leave it to stand until all the water is completely absorbed. Segment the orange and squeeze the juice from the peel and membrane over the couscous. Set the orange segments aside for later and fluff up the couscous with a fork.

To cook the cauliflower and broccoli, bring a pan of water to the boil and add salt. Add the cauliflower and broccoli to the pan, blanch for 2 minutes, then drain and refresh under cold water.

Heat the olive oil in a wide frying pan. When it's hot, add the cauliflower and broccoli and sauté over a high heat, stirring regularly. When brown patches start to appear, add the chickpeas, baharat spice and garlic. Cook for another couple of minutes, so the vegetables and chickpeas are well coated with the spice, then remove the pan from the heat and leave the veg to cool to room temperature.

Make the dressing. Whisk everything together and season with salt and pepper.

To assemble, sprinkle the couscous over a large platter and top with the spinach leaves, followed by the cauliflower, broccoli and chickpeas. Drain the onion and raisins and sprinkle them on top, then drizzle over the salad dressing.

Add the herbs, orange segments and flaked almonds, and finish with a generous sprinkling of sumac.

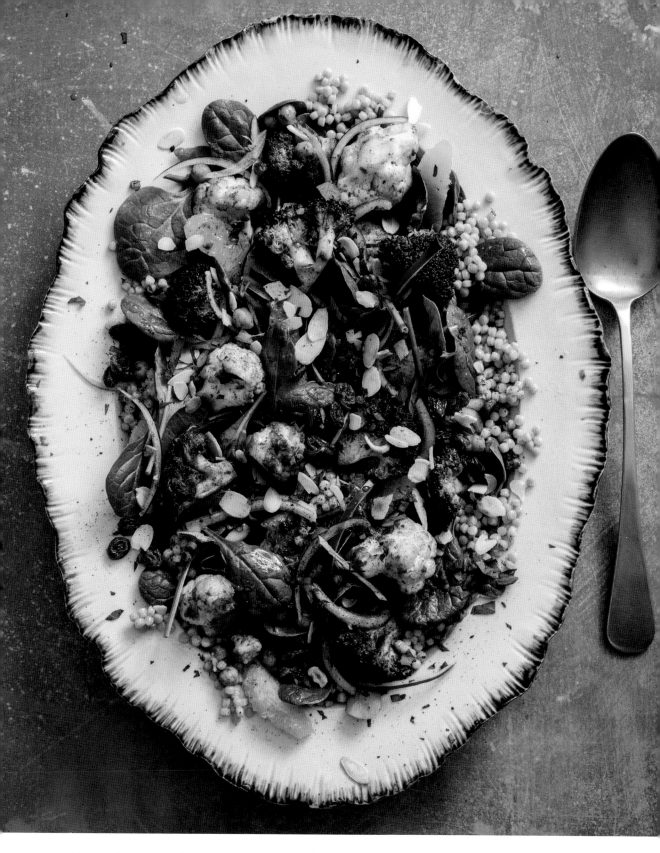

INFO PER SERVING: PROTEIN (G) 15   CARBS (G) 40   SUGAR (G) 19   FAT (G) 20.5   SATURATED FAT (G) 3   FIBRE (G) 11.5   SALT (G) 0.1

Serves: **4**

 Prep: **10 minutes**

 Cooking time:
about 30 minutes

 Calories per serving:
420

ROAST CARROT & RED CABBAGE SALAD

750g carrots, trimmed

1 small red cabbage, cut into
   slim wedges

3 tbsp olive oil

250g halloumi, cut into slices
   and patted dry

1 tsp dried mint

100g baby spinach

a few fresh mint leaves

2–3 tsp za'atar

salt and black pepper

DRESSING

1 tbsp tahini

juice of 1 lemon

1 tsp honey

1 small garlic clove, crushed
   or grated

You could make this salad with just the carrots, halloumi and spinach leaves but it's even better with the addition of some wedges of cabbage. Red cabbage looks lovely, but you could also use the green pointed kind if you prefer. We're loving za'atar by the way. It's a Middle Eastern spice mix that adds a lovely flavour to dishes and it's available in supermarkets.

Preheat the oven to 200°C/Fan 180°C/Gas 6.

Cut the carrots into even-sized lengths and put them in a roasting tray with the red cabbage wedges. Drizzle over 2 tablespoons of the olive oil and toss until everything is evenly coated. Season with salt and pepper. Roast for about 25 minutes, turning the veg over a couple of times, until lightly browned and tender to the point of a knife. Remove from the oven and leave to cool.

Heat the remaining olive oil in a frying pan. Add the slices of halloumi and fry them until well browned on both sides. Remove the slices from the frying pan and roughly chop, then sprinkle with the dried mint.

Make the salad dressing. Whisk all the ingredients together and season with plenty of salt and pepper. Thin with just enough water to make a pourable consistency.

Toss the carrots and cabbage with the halloumi and spinach. Drizzle over the dressing and sprinkle over the mint leaves and the za'atar before serving.

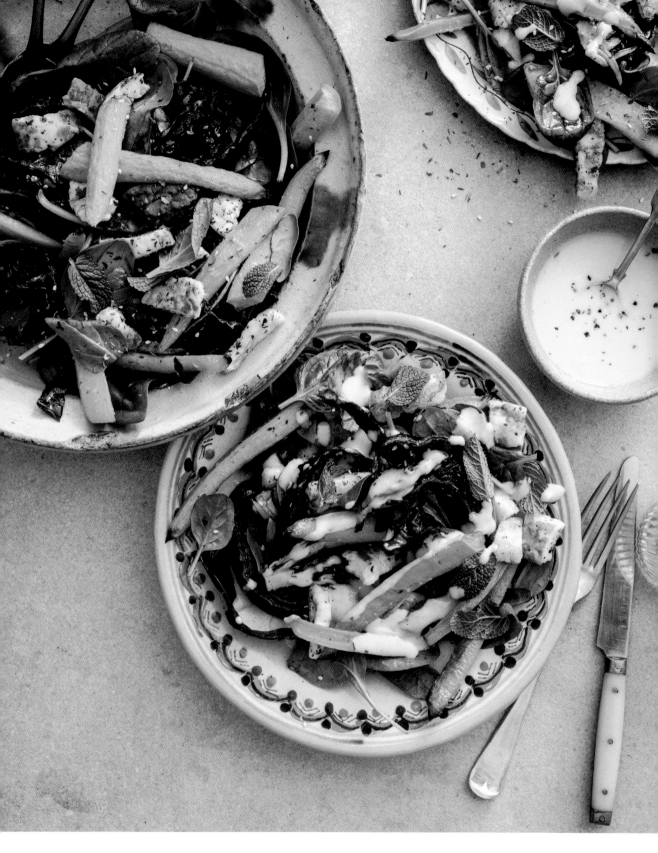

INFO PER SERVING: PROTEIN (G) 19   CARBS (G) 20   SUGAR (G) 18.5   FAT (G) 27   SATURATED FAT (G) 12   FIBRE (G) 12   SALT (G) 2

Serves: **4**

 Prep: **10 minutes**

 Cooking time:
about 15 minutes

 Calories per serving:
344

PUTTANESCA-STYLE PASTA SALAD

250g short pasta, such as
penne or fusilli

125g wild rocket, roughly
chopped

300g cherry tomatoes,
chopped

50g pitted olives, sliced
(green or black)

50g capers, rinsed

½ tsp chilli flakes

leaves from 2 basil sprigs,
roughly torn

25g Parmesan, shaved

salt and black pepper

DRESSING

30g can of anchovies
and their oil

1 tbsp olive oil

zest and juice of 1 lemon

2 garlic cloves, crushed

leaves from a thyme sprig
or ½ tsp dried thyme

Pasta salads can be a bit boring but try our new fiery and flavourful version and we're sure you'll be converted. Puttanesca, one of the classic Italian sauces, is a great favourite of ours and here we're using some of the same ingredients, such as chilli flakes, capers and olives, to make a really exciting salad.

First make the dressing. Put the anchovies in a small saucepan with the olive oil. Heat gently, breaking up the anchovies with the back of a spoon until they start to dissolve into the oil. Add the lemon zest and juice, followed by the garlic and thyme. Season with black pepper. Cook very gently – don't let the garlic take on any colour – then remove the pan from the heat and set aside.

Cook the pasta in plenty of salted, boiling water. When it's al dente, drain, tip it into a bowl and immediately pour the dressing over it. Toss to combine and leave the pasta to cool until it's just about at room temperature.

Add the rocket, tomatoes, olives, capers and chilli flakes. Mix thoroughly, then lightly toss with the basil leaves. Serve with shavings of Parmesan.

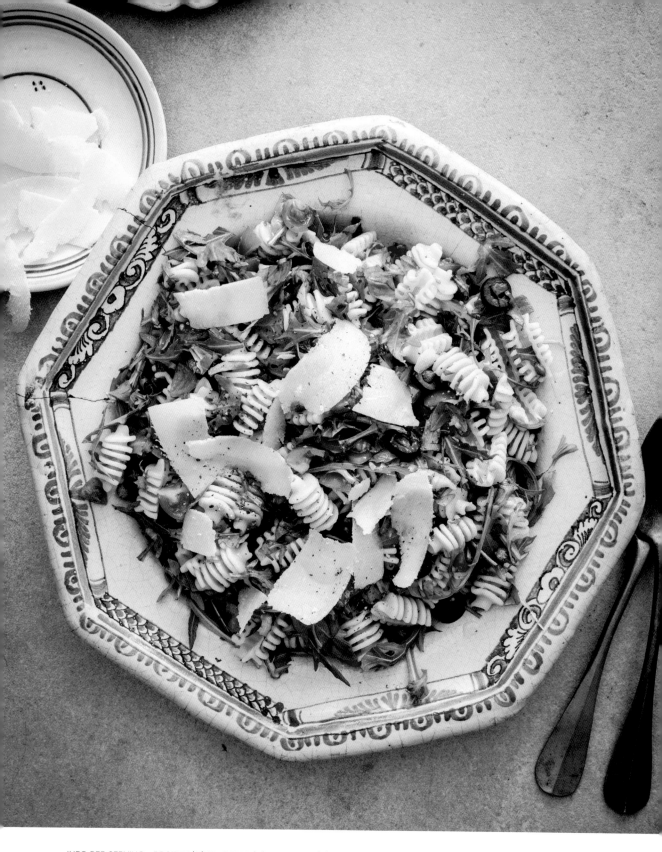

INFO PER SERVING: PROTEIN (G) 14   CARBS (G) 49   SUGAR (G) 4   FAT (G) 9   SATURATED FAT (G) 2   FIBRE (G) 5   SALT (G) 1.8

Serves: **4**

 Prep: **10 minutes**

 Cooking time:
no cooking

 Calories per serving:
400

WHITE BEAN & TUNA SALAD

2 x 400g cans of cannellini
    beans, drained
200g canned or jarred tuna
    (or use 2 x 160g cans, each
    112g drained weight)
100g black pitted olives,
    roughly chopped
100g rocket, roughly chopped
2 heads of red chicory or
    1 radicchio, shredded
100g cherry tomatoes
1 small red onion, finely sliced
a few thyme and/or basil
    leaves

DRESSING
2 tbsp olive oil
juice and zest of ½ lemon
1 tsp sherry vinegar
2 tsp Dijon or wholegrain
    mustard
leaves from 2 tarragon sprigs,
    finely chopped
salt and black pepper

When you want an appetising meal in a hurry, try this recipe – it uses mostly store-cupboard ingredients and you'll have a whole meal in a bowl in no time. The red chicory or radicchio does add a nice touch of bitterness and vibrant colour but if you can't find any, use any salad leaves you like.

First make the dressing. Whisk everything together and season with salt and pepper.

Put all the salad ingredients in a bowl and drizzle over the salad dressing. Mix gently but thoroughly, then divide between 4 bowls.

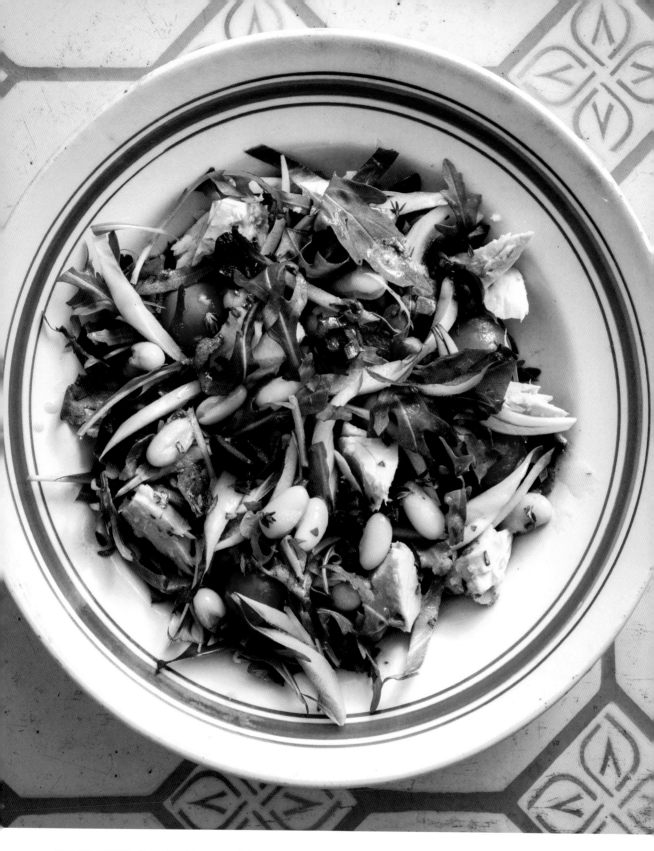

INFO PER SERVING: PROTEIN (G) 26 CARBS (G) 29 SUGAR (G) 3 FAT (G) 17.5 SATURATED FAT (G) 2.5 FIBRE (G) 11.5 SALT (G) 1.5

Serves: **4**

 Prep: **15 minutes, plus standing time**

 Cooking time: **about 10 minutes**

 Calories: **258**

SQUID, PRAWN & BLACK BEAN SALAD

300g sprouting broccoli

200g squid rings

200g raw prawns (shelled weight)

400g can of black beans, drained

1 red pepper, diced

1 mango, peeled and diced

50g micro or salad leaves

small bunch of coriander, roughly chopped

DRESSING

zest and juice of 2 limes

2 tsp chilli paste or hot sauce (any sort)

1 garlic clove, finely chopped

1 tbsp olive oil

2 tsp red wine vinegar

¼ tsp ground cinnamon

1 red onion, thinly sliced

salt and black pepper

Squid should be cooked either long and slow or short and fast and for this recipe it needs just a minute in the pan. Lots of interesting flavours and textures in this salad and it looks beautiful too. Just be sure your mango is not too ripe, as you want to be able to dice it neatly.

Mix all the dressing ingredients together in a large bowl, season with salt and pepper and leave to stand for half an hour.

Bring a large pan of water to a rolling boil. Add the sprouting broccoli and cook for 3–4 minutes until just tender. Remove the broccoli from the pan with a slotted spoon and set it aside, then bring the water back to the boil. Add the squid and cook for 60 seconds. Remove the squid from the pan with a slotted spoon and then add the prawns. Cook until they are pink, then remove.

Add the cooked broccoli, squid and prawns to the dressing and leave until they are at room temperature. Add the remaining ingredients and gently fold everything together. Leave the salad to stand for 5 minutes to allow the flavours to blend a little, then divide between 4 bowls and serve.

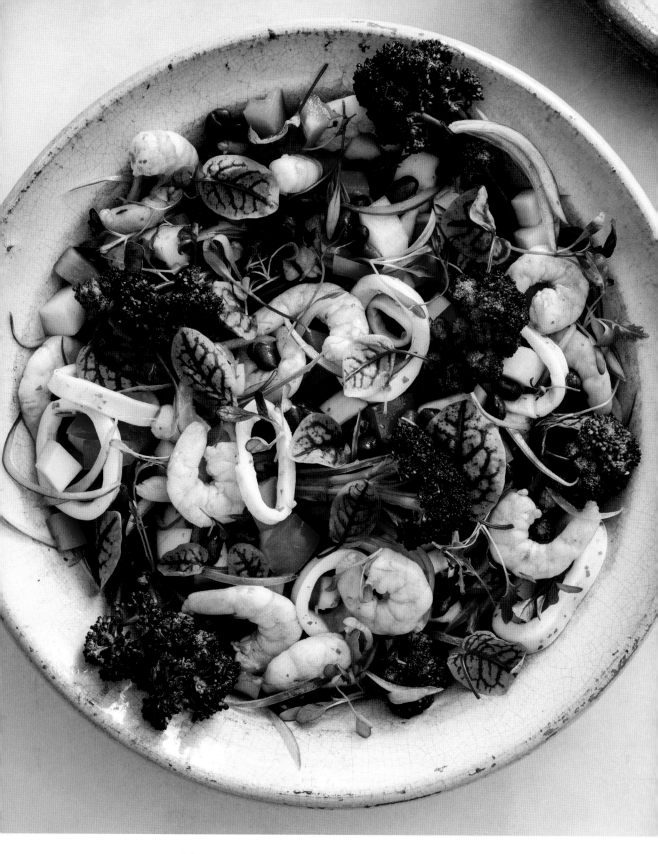

INFO PER SERVING: PROTEIN (G) 26   CARBS (G) 22.5   SUGAR (G) 11   FAT (G) 5.5   SATURATED FAT (G) 1   FIBRE (G) 9   SALT (G) 0.6

Serves: **4**

 Prep: **15 minutes, plus marinating**

 Cooking time: **up to 35 minutes**

 Calories per serving: **470**

CHICKEN & FREEKEH SALAD

400g skinless, boneless chicken breast or thigh meat
100g plain yoghurt
1 tbsp sumac
zest of 1 lemon
1 tbsp za'atar
1 tbsp olive oil
salt and black pepper

FREEKEH
100g cracked freekeh (or 250–300g ready-cooked)
1 tbsp olive oil
1 tsp ground allspice

DRESSING
1 tbsp tahini
1 tbsp olive oil
juice of 1 lemon
1 tsp red wine vinegar
1 tsp honey

TO ASSEMBLE
50g lamb's lettuce
½ cucumber, deseeded and sliced into crescents
3 apricots, stoned and cut into wedges
a few mint leaves

Very popular in Middle Eastern countries, freekeh is a kind of wheat that is picked while still green and soft, then roasted. It can be used in the same way as couscous and bulgur and is high in fibre and very nutritious. It's got a great nutty taste too that goes beautifully with the chicken and other ingredients in this salad.

Preheat the oven to 200°C/Fan 180°C/Gas 6. Line a baking tray with baking parchment. Slice the chicken into strips and season them with salt and pepper. Mix the yoghurt with the sumac and lemon zest in a bowl, then add the chicken. Stir well to combine, then leave to marinate for half an hour.

Arrange the chicken strips on a baking tray, well spaced apart, then sprinkle over the za'atar and drizzle over the oil. Bake in the oven for about 12 minutes, until cooked through and lightly browned. Set aside.

If cooking the freekeh, wash it thoroughly and soak it in a bowl of water for 10 minutes, then drain thoroughly. Heat the olive oil in a saucepan and add the freekeh. Toast in the oil until the nutty, smoky aroma becomes quite pronounced, then stir in the allspice. Season with salt and black pepper, then add 300ml of water. Bring to the boil, then turn down the heat and cover. Leave to cook for 15–20 minutes until the freekeh is tender and all the liquid has been absorbed. (If using ready-cooked freekeh, put it in a bowl and stir in the oil and allspice.)

To make the dressing, whisk the ingredients together and season with salt and pepper. If necessary, add a little water to thin the dressing out.

To assemble, arrange the freekeh, lamb's lettuce and cucumber on a serving dish and drizzle over some of the dressing. Top with the apricots and chicken strips. Drizzle over more of the salad dressing and top with a few mint leaves. Add another sprinkling of sumac and za'atar if you like.

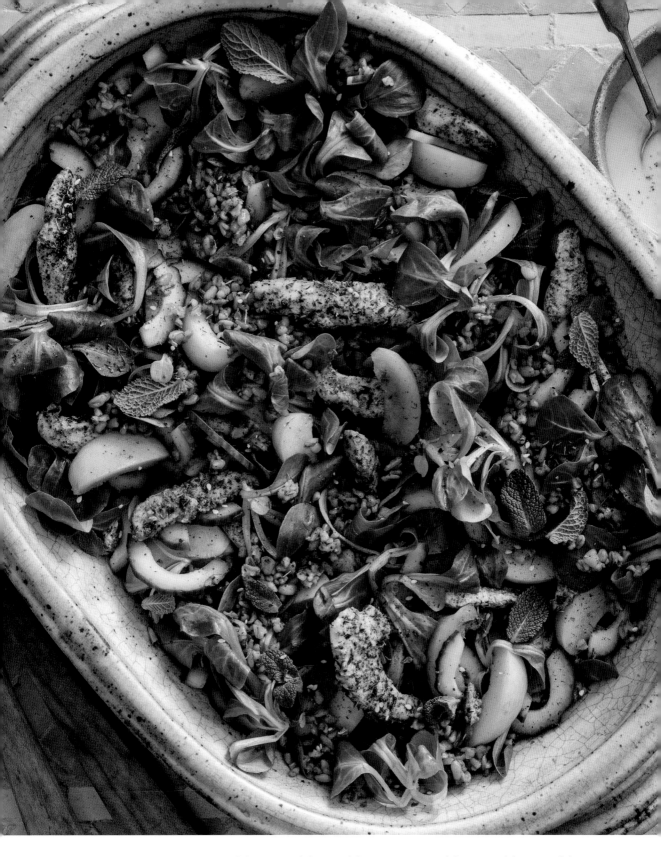

INFO PER SERVING: PROTEIN (G) 36   CARBS (G) 42   SUGAR (G) 26   FAT (G) 15   SATURATED FAT (G) 2.5   FIBRE (G) 11.5   SALT (G) 0.5

Serves: **4**

 Prep: **15 minutes**

 Cooking time:
up to 10 minutes, plus resting time

 Calories per serving:
266

GRILLED BEEF & BEETROOT SALAD

400g steak (bavette, onglet or minute are the cheapest), at room temperature

125g mixed leaves – the one with beet leaves is good

100g cooked spelt

2 heads of chicory, broken up and roughly chopped

250g beetroot, cut into wedges (vac-packed are fine)

leaves from a small bunch of parsley, roughly chopped

seeds from ½ pomegranate

salt and black pepper

SALAD DRESSING

2 tbsp olive oil

2 shallots, finely sliced

1 tbsp red wine vinegar

½ tsp mixed herbs or dried thyme

1 tsp Dijon or tarragon mustard

Beef and beetroot go beautifully together in this substantial and very special salad. We like bavette steak, as it's full of flavour and not as expensive as some cuts. For speed, we decided to use ready-cooked spelt, available in sachets, but cook your own if you prefer, or choose another grain such as barley. Pomegranate seeds add a bit of sharp sweetness and crunch to this cracking dish.

Make sure the steak is at room temperature – remove it from the fridge about half an hour before cooking. Sprinkle with plenty of salt and black pepper.

Heat a griddle until it's too hot to hold your hand over for more than a few seconds, then add the steak. Leave the steak without turning it for several minutes until it can be lifted off the griddle cleanly and has deep char lines. Turn and cook the other side for several minutes, again until it will lift off cleanly. This will give you a steak between rare and medium rare, depending on how thick it is. If you like your steak medium-rare to medium, cook for another 2–3 minutes on each side.

Transfer the steak to a board and leave it to rest for at least 10 minutes. Pour any juices that drain from the steak into a bowl.

Whisk all the dressing ingredients together and add the steak juices. Taste for seasoning and add salt and pepper as necessary.

Assemble the salad. Arrange the mixed leaves over a large serving dish and sprinkle over the spelt. Drizzle over a little of the dressing, then add the chicory and beetroot. Thinly slice the beef and add this too, then pour over the remaining dressing. Finish with the parsley leaves and pomegranate seeds, then serve.

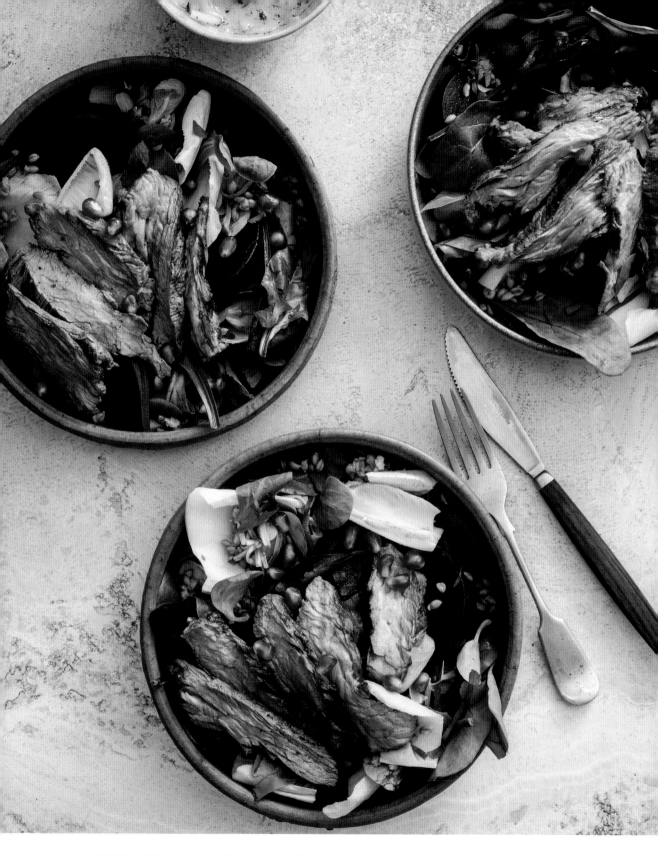

INFO PER SERVING: PROTEIN (G) 25   CARBS (G) 16   SUGAR (G) 8   FAT (G) 10   SATURATED FAT (G) 2.5   FIBRE (G) 4   SALT (G) 0.4

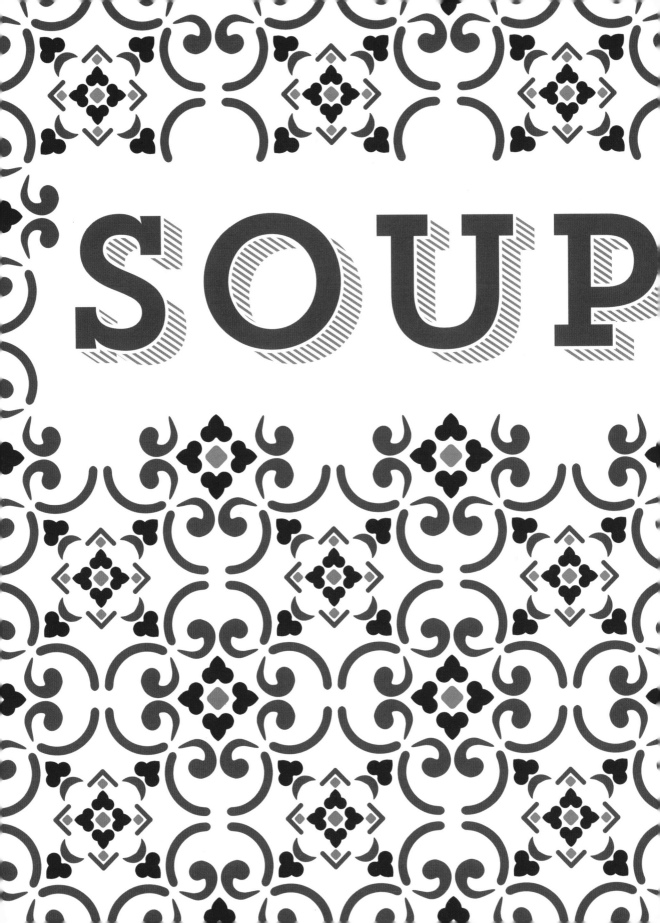

WATERCRESS, POTATO
& LEMON SOUP

COURGETTE &
YOGHURT SOUP

MUSHROOM & BARLEY
SOUP

TOMATO, GINGER &
RICE SOUP

LENTIL, SQUASH &
KALE SOUP

CARROT & SWEET
POTATO SOUP

BLACK BEAN &
VEGETABLE SOUP

CHICKEN & WHITE
BEAN SOUP

Serves: **4**

 Prep: **10 minutes**

 Cooking time:
about 30 minutes

 Calories per serving:
123

WATERCRESS, POTATO & LEMON SOUP

1 tbsp olive oil

5g butter

1 onion, finely chopped

1 leek, finely chopped
(optional)

150g potato, skin on, finely
diced

75g celeriac, peeled and finely
diced

2 garlic cloves, finely chopped

150g watercress

zest and juice of ½ lemon

800ml vegetable or chicken
stock or water

freshly grated nutmeg

salt and black pepper

With its great punchy, peppery flavour, watercress makes a tasty soup or you could also use one of those mixed bags of watercress, rocket and spinach. We've cut down on the amount of potato and included some celeriac which has a good flavour and is lower in calories – also ups your veg count which is always a good plan.

Heat the olive oil and butter in a saucepan. When the butter has melted, add the onion, leek, if using, potato and celeriac and stir until they are all coated with the oil and butter. Season with salt and pepper. Cover the pan and leave the vegetables to sweat for up to 10 minutes, stirring gently until they are just cooked through, then stir in the chopped garlic.

Separate the watercress leaves from the stems. Roughly chop the stems and stir them into the vegetables. Add the lemon zest and pour the stock or water into the pan, then bring to the boil and simmer until everything is tender.

Add the watercress leaves, reserving a few to use as a garnish, and let them wilt into the soup for a moment. Blitz the soup until smooth – a little green flecking is good. Add the lemon juice and taste for seasoning. Serve the soup topped with a rasp of nutmeg and garnished with a few watercress leaves.

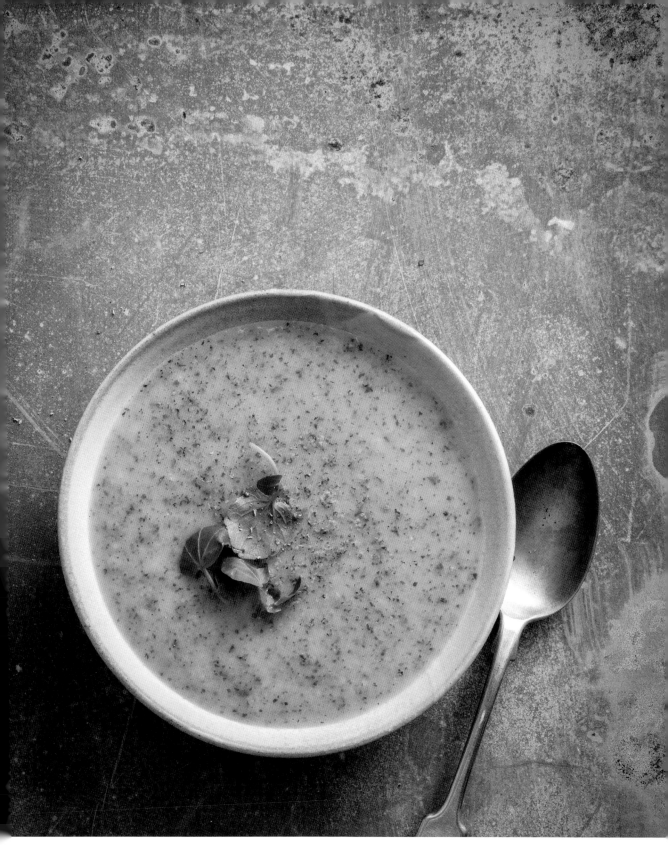

INFO PER SERVING: PROTEIN (G) 4   CARBS (G) 13   SUGAR (G) 5   FAT (G) 5   SATURATED FAT (G) 1.5   FIBRE (G) 5   SALT (G) 0.4

Serves: **4**

 Prep: **10 minutes**

 Cooking time: **about 30 minutes**

 Calories per serving with topping/without: **215/135**

COURGETTE & YOGHURT SOUP

1 tbsp olive oil

1 small onion, finely chopped

1 leek, sliced

2 large courgettes (about 400g), sliced

3 garlic cloves, finely chopped

1 tsp dried mint

zest and juice of 1 lime

25g red lentils

750ml vegetable or chicken stock

100g Greek yoghurt or kefir

salt and black pepper

TOPPING (OPTIONAL)

2 tsp olive oil

3 tbsp pumpkin seeds

Soups of this sort usually need some kind of thickener which tends to be rice, potatoes or flour, but we're using a small amount of lentils here instead. They're better for you and work just as well, if not better, for thickening the soup. Velvety and scrumptious.

Heat the oil in a large saucepan. Add the onion and leek and sauté them over a low heat until translucent. Add the courgettes and garlic and stir for another couple of minutes, then add the dried mint, lime zest and red lentils.

Pour in the stock and season with salt and pepper. Bring to the boil, then turn down the heat and cover the pan. Simmer until the vegetables are tender and the lentils have started to disintegrate – about 15 minutes.

For the garnish, if using, heat the olive oil in a small frying pan and add the pumpkin seeds. Stir-fry until they smell toasted.

Purée the soup with a stick or jug blender until quite smooth and flecked with green. Add the yoghurt or kefir and stir it in until completely combined. Heat the soup very gently – you don't want the yoghurt to separate – then stir in the lime juice. If using the garnish, sprinkle some on top of each serving.

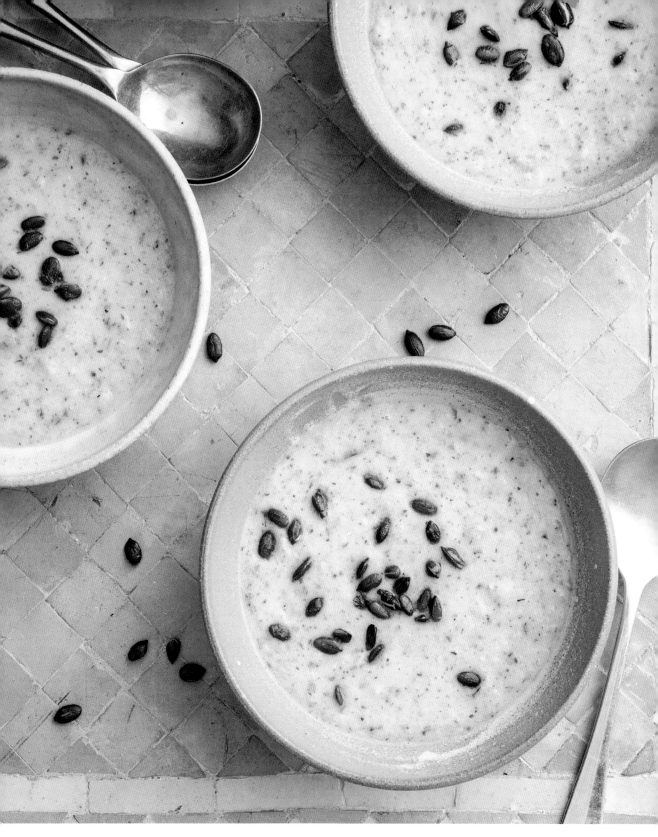

INFO PER SERVING WITH TOPPING/WITHOUT: PROTEIN (G) 9.5/6 CARBS (G) 12/10.5 SUGAR (G) 6.5/6.5 FAT (G) 13/6.5

SATURATED FAT (G) 3.5/2.5 FIBRE (G) 5/4 SALT (G) 0.2/0.2

Serves: **4**

 Prep: **15 minutes**

 Cooking time:
about 40 minutes

 Calories per serving
with bacon/without:
327/240

MUSHROOM & BARLEY SOUP

200g cooked barley
(about 50g uncooked)

1 tbsp olive oil

1 small onion, finely chopped

1 leek, finely sliced

400g mushrooms, sliced

2 tsp mustard powder

2 garlic cloves, chopped

leaves from a thyme sprig

leaves from 2 tarragon sprigs,
finely chopped

15g dried mushrooms, soaked
in warm water

100g kale, destemmed and
finely chopped

1 litre mushroom stock

75g crème fraiche

salt and black pepper

TO SERVE (OPTIONAL)
4 slices of bacon, fried and
crumbled

Barley is an excellent grain to add to your diet, as it's high in fibre and rich in vitamins and minerals. For this hearty soup, it's best to cook the barley separately, as the cooking time can vary quite a bit. The mustard powder provides just the right amount of body for the soup – the texture isn't like a broth, but it isn't thick either. A real winter warmer.

Cook the barley according to the packet instructions and set aside.

Heat the olive oil in a large saucepan. Add the onion, leek and fresh mushrooms. Sauté over a medium-high heat until the mushrooms have collapsed down and the base of the pan looks quite dry, then stir in the mustard powder, garlic and herbs.

Drain the dried mushrooms, reserving their soaking liquor. Chop them finely and add them to the pan along with the kale. Strain the soaking liquor to remove any grit, then add this to the pan with the stock. Season with salt and pepper.

Bring to the boil, then turn the heat down and simmer the soup for about 15 minutes until the vegetables are completely tender. Stir in the barley and crème fraiche and heat through for a few more minutes – don't let the soup come to the boil.

Serve as is or with the bacon garnish.

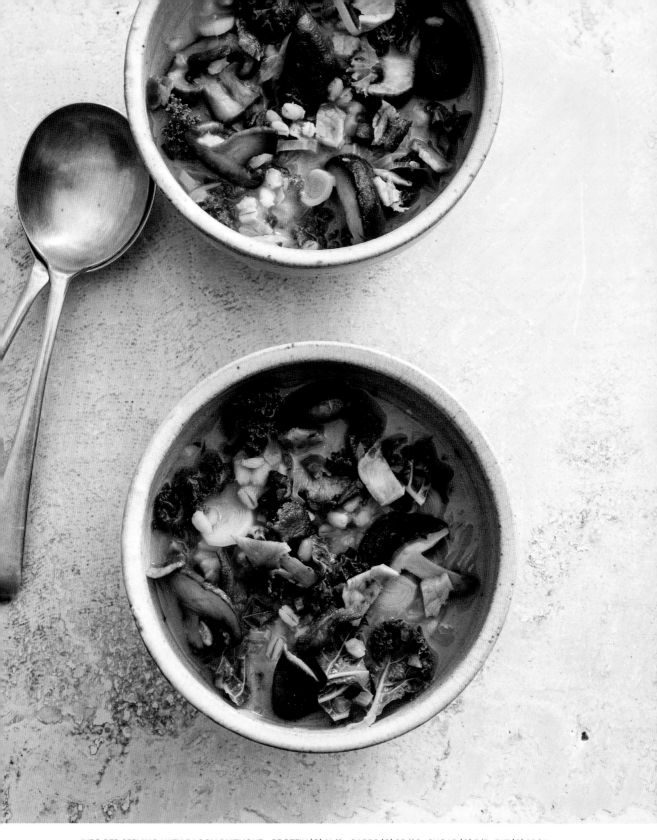

INFO PER SERVING WITH BACON/WITHOUT: PROTEIN (G) 14/8   CARBS (G) 20/20   SUGAR (G) 5/5   FAT (G) 20/13

SATURATED FAT (G) 8.5/6   FIBRE (G) 5/5   SALT (G) 1/0.2

Serves: **4**

 Prep: **10 minutes**

 Cooking time:
about 30 minutes

 Calories per serving:
143

TOMATO, GINGER & RICE SOUP

1 tsp coconut oil

a few curry leaves

3 shallots or 1 onion, finely
   sliced

5g root ginger, finely chopped

3 garlic cloves, finely chopped

2 tsp ground cumin

1 tsp chilli powder

500g fresh tomatoes, roughly
   chopped or puréed

1 tbsp tamarind paste

750ml vegetable stock or
   water

pinch of ground cinnamon
   (optional)

½ tsp honey or sugar (optional)

2 tsp garam masala

100g wholegrain black or wild
   rice, cooked according to
   the packet instructions

leaves from a small bunch of
   coriander (optional)

salt and black pepper

Who doesn't love a tomato soup? And we hope you'll agree that this recipe, enriched with rice and spice, is a real keeper. We suggest using fresh tomatoes for the best results but if necessary you could use canned. Both black and wild rice have a lovely nutty flavour which is good here, and if you want to use ready-cooked rice you'll need about 220g.

Heat the coconut oil in a large saucepan. Add the curry leaves and fry until they start to crackle, then add the shallots or onion. Fry for a few minutes until the shallots or onion are starting to take on some colour, then stir in the ginger, garlic and spices. Stir well until everything smells very aromatic, then add the tomatoes.

Cook the tomatoes over a medium-high heat, stirring regularly, until they start to look a little jammy, then season with salt and pepper. Add the tamarind paste and stock or water. Bring to the boil, then turn down the heat and simmer for about 15 minutes. Taste the soup and if it seems a little sour for your taste, add a pinch of cinnamon and/or the honey or sugar. Stir to combine, then stir in the garam masala.

Serve the soup in bowls and stir some rice into each serving. Garnish with fresh coriander leaves, if using.

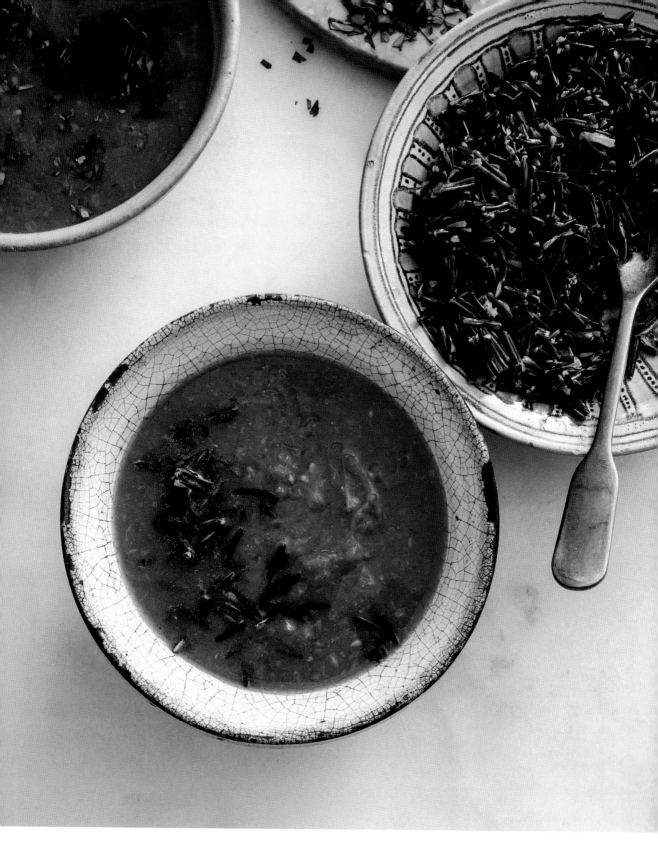

INFO PER SERVING: PROTEIN (G) 3   CARBS (G) 25   SUGAR (G) 6.5   FAT (G) 2.5   SATURATED FAT (G) 1.5   FIBRE (G) 3   SALT (G) 0.1

Serves: **4**

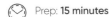 Prep: **15 minutes**

Cooking time:
about 40 minutes

 Calories per serving
with toppings/without:
235/205

LENTIL, SQUASH & KALE SOUP

1 tbsp olive oil

1 red onion, diced

300g squash, peeled and
   diced

3 garlic cloves, finely chopped

2 tsp baharat spice mix

100g brown or green lentils

about 1 litre vegetable or
   chicken stock

200g kale, shredded

200g passata or chopped
   tomatoes

juice of ½ lemon

salt and black pepper

TOPPING (OPTIONAL)

150g yoghurt or kefir

1 tsp dried mint

1 tbsp preserved lemon, finely
   chopped

a few fresh mint leaves

Make this as a chunky soup or a veggie stew, depending on how much liquid you add – it's a winner either way and is a good filling meal. We suggest making a little yoghurt and preserved lemon topping to add extra zing, or you could just stir in some chopped preserved lemon and garnish with mint and perhaps a bit of crumbled feta. Whatever takes your fancy.

Heat the olive oil in a large saucepan. Add the onion and sauté it over a medium heat until it starts to take on some colour. Add the squash and garlic, and continue to cook for another 2–3 minutes, before stirring in the baharat spice, then the lentils.

Pour in the stock and season with salt and pepper, then bring to the boil and partially cover the pan. Leave to cook at a reasonably fast boil for 15 minutes, then test the lentils – they should be well on their way to being cooked at this point. Push the kale into the stock, then add the passata or tomatoes.

Continue to simmer the soup, partially covered, until the lentils and kale are tender. This will probably take another 20 minutes, but start testing after 15. Taste and adjust the seasoning as necessary and add the lemon juice.

If making the topping, mix the yoghurt or kefir with the dried mint and preserved lemon, then season with salt and pepper and sprinkle with a few fresh mint leaves. Serve the garnish at the table so everyone can add a dollop to their bowl.

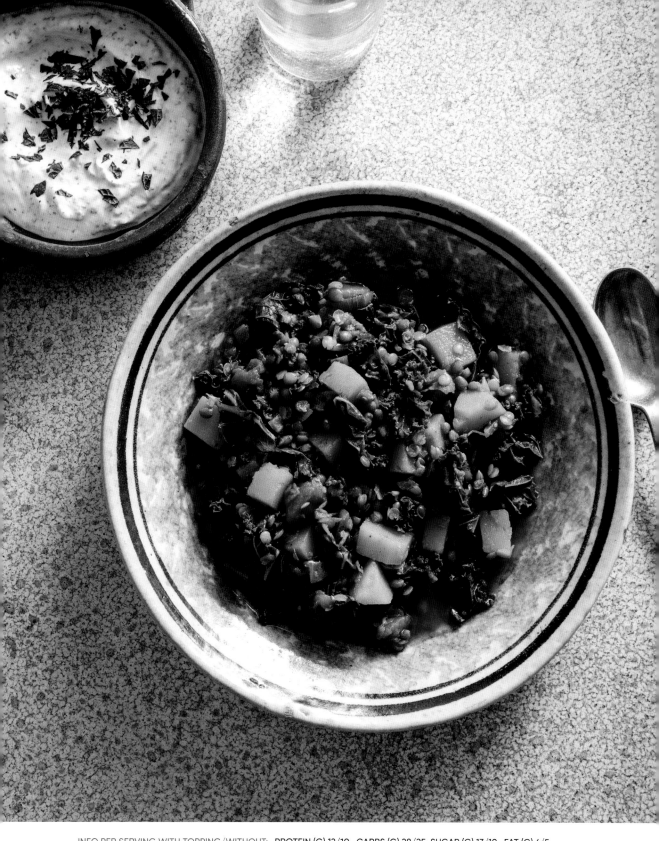

INFO PER SERVING WITH TOPPING/WITHOUT: PROTEIN (G) 12/10   CARBS (G) 28/25   SUGAR (G) 13/10   FAT (G) 6/5

SATURATED FAT (G) 2/1   FIBRE (G) 9/9   SALT (G) 0.5/0.2

Serves: **4**

 Prep: **10 minutes**

 Cooking time:
about 20 minutes

 Calories per serving:
208

CARROT & SWEET POTATO SOUP

1 tbsp olive oil

1 onion, finely chopped

400g carrots, diced

1 sweet potato, diced

2 garlic cloves, finely chopped

5g root ginger, finely chopped

800ml vegetable stock or
    dashi

1–2 tbsp miso

1 tbsp tamari or dark soy sauce

2 tbsp freshly squeezed orange
    juice

salt and black pepper

TOPPINGS

2 spring onions, very finely
    sliced into rounds

2 tsp sesame oil

1 tsp black sesame seeds

Rich in colour and flavour, this is a simple soup to make and a cracking good eat. Enjoy with a sprinkle of spring onions and sesame oil and seeds for extra flavour and nutrients.

Heat the oil in a large saucepan. Add the onion, carrots and sweet potato. Sauté over a high heat until the vegetables are starting to take on some colour around the edges, then add the garlic and ginger. Stir for another couple of minutes.

Pour in the stock and season with salt and black pepper. Simmer for about another 10 minutes until the vegetables are completely tender.

Stir in a tablespoon of the miso, then the tamari or soy sauce and the orange juice. Purée the soup with a stick or jug blender and taste, then add more miso if you think it necessary. Heat the soup through again until piping hot.

Ladle into bowls and sprinkle over the spring onions, sesame oil and seeds.

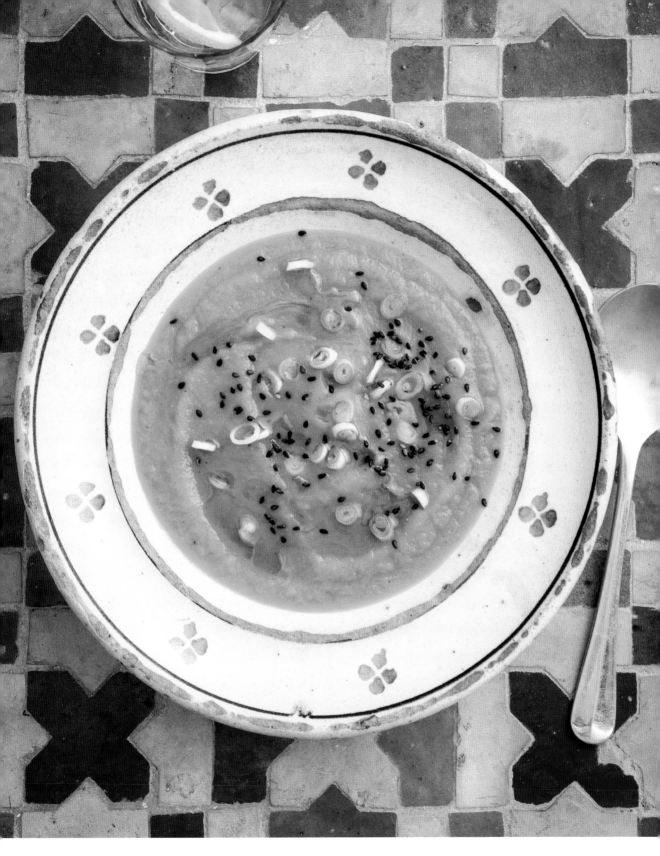

INFO PER SERVING: PROTEIN (G) 3.5   CARBS (G) 27   SUGAR (G) 15   FAT (G) 8   SATURATED FAT (G) 1.5   FIBRE (G) 7   SALT (G) 1

Serves: **4**

 Prep: **10 minutes**

Cooking time:
about 30 minutes

 Calories per serving:
429

BLACK BEAN & VEGETABLE SOUP

1 tbsp olive oil

1 onion, diced

1 red pepper, diced

200g butternut squash, diced

3 garlic cloves, finely chopped

1 tsp ground cumin

½ tsp ground cinnamon

1 tsp chilli paste or powder

2 tbsp tomato purée

2 bay leaves

2 x 400g cans of black beans, drained

200g sweetcorn (frozen is best)

400ml can of coconut milk

400ml vegetable stock

4 cubes of frozen spinach

salt and black pepper

TO SERVE

1 large avocado, diced

juice of 1 lime

small bunch of coriander, finely chopped (optional)

A lovely robust soup, this one is great for making sure you get your five-a-day. Black beans are readily available and are particularly high in protein and fibre, so you'll be doing yourself good as well as enjoying a taste treat.

Heat the olive oil in a large saucepan and add the onion, red pepper and squash. Sauté over a high heat until the vegetables have started to soften, then stir in the garlic. Cook for a further 2 minutes.

Stir in the spices and chilli paste or powder, followed by the tomato purée. Add the bay leaves, black beans and sweetcorn, then pour in the coconut milk and stock. Stir well to make sure the base of the pan is clean, then season with salt and pepper. Drop in the cubes of spinach.

Bring to the boil, then turn down the heat, cover the pan and leave to simmer for about 20 minutes until the vegetables are tender.

Toss the avocado in the lime juice and serve with the soup. Sprinkle with fresh coriander, if using.

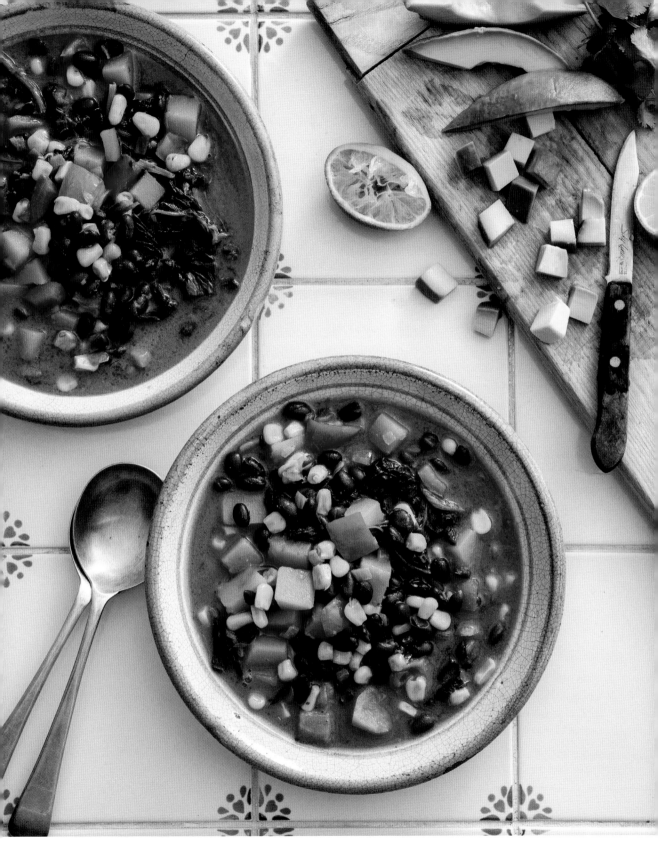

INFO PER SERVING: PROTEIN (G) 14.5   CARBS (G) 38   SUGAR (G) 11.5   FAT (G) 22   SATURATED FAT (G) 15.5   FIBRE (G) 10   SALT (G) 0.3

Serves: **4**

 Prep: **15 minutes**

 Cooking time:
about 25 minutes

 Calories per serving:
472

CHICKEN & WHITE BEAN SOUP

1 tbsp olive oil

1 small onion, finely chopped

2 leeks, sliced into rounds

2 medium courgettes, sliced
   on the diagonal

250g broccoli, sliced into
   florets

3 garlic cloves, finely chopped

2 bay leaves

1 large tarragon sprig

piece of pared lemon zest

100ml white wine

2 x 400g cans of cannellini
   beans, drained

800ml chicken stock

about 400g cooked, skinless
   chicken breast meat,
   shredded

salt and black pepper

PESTO

25g basil leaves

25g ground almonds

zest of 1 lemon

1 garlic clove, finely chopped

1 tbsp olive oil

Chicken soup is a real comforting hug of a dish and this great version is packed with veggies and served topped with a quick pesto. Use ready-cooked chicken breasts or some that you have leftover from a Sunday roast. Get chopping and enjoy!

Heat the olive oil in a large saucepan and add the onion. Sauté for a few minutes until it's starting to turn translucent, then add the leeks, courgettes, broccoli, garlic, herbs and lemon zest. Stir to combine and season with salt and pepper. Pour over the wine and leave it to bubble up for a minute, then turn down the heat, cover the pan and leave to cook for 8–10 minutes until the vegetables are tender.

Roughly mash about a third of the beans to add texture to the soup, then add them all – mashed and whole – to the vegetables. Pour in the chicken stock and bring to the boil. When the soup is piping hot, taste for seasoning. Add the chicken and leave it to heat through for a few moments.

While the soup is cooking, make the pesto. Put everything into a food processor and blitz to form a paste, then season with salt and pepper. Serve the soup with spoonfuls of the pesto to swirl through it.

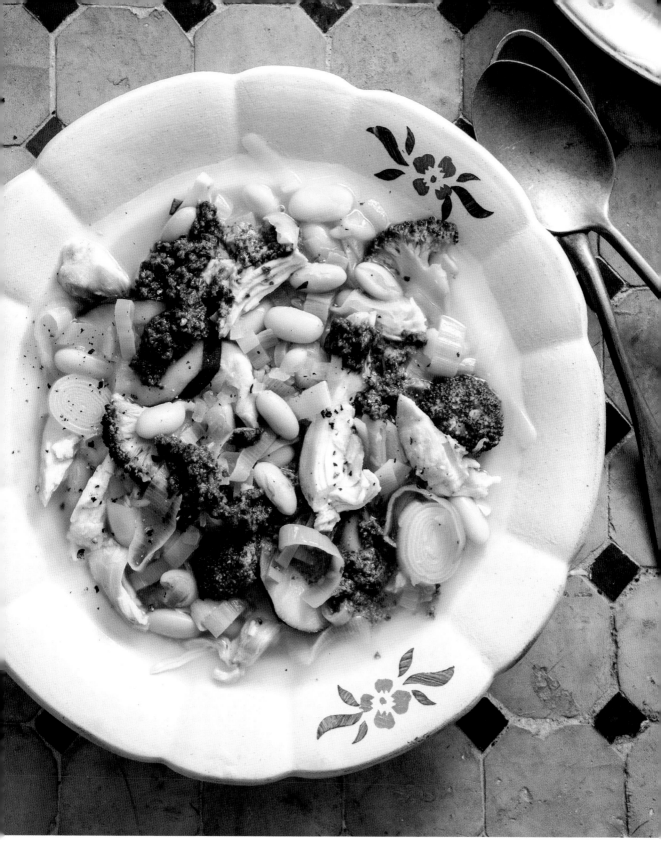

INFO PER SERVING: PROTEIN (G) 45   CARBS (G) 30   SUGAR (G) 7   FAT (G) 14   SATURATED FAT (G) 2.5   FIBRE (G) 16   SALT (G) 0.4

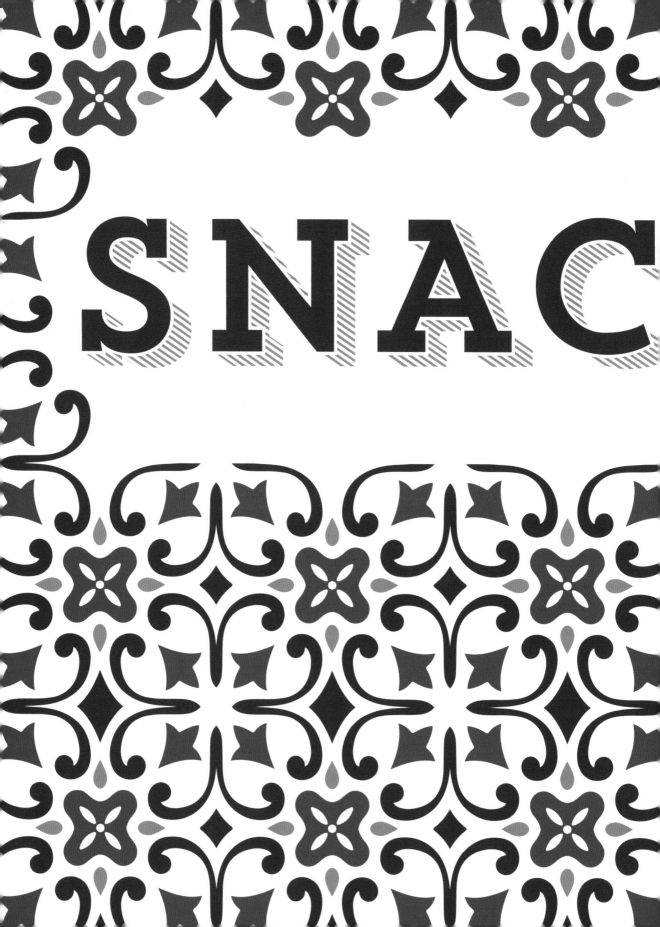

K S

FIG & WALNUT CRACKERS

BLACK BREAD WITH SEEDS

DELICIOUS DIPS

TOMATO & RICOTTA TOAST TOPPER

FLATBREADS WITH TURMERIC & BLACK PEPPER

LENTIL & ALMOND PÂTÉ

TOFU WITH TOMATO & AVOCADO

VEGETABLE FRITTERS

CHOCOLATE & TAHINI ENERGY BOMBS

Makes: **about 30**

 Prep: **10 minutes**

 Cooking time:
about 1 hour 10 minutes, plus cooling

 Calories per cracker: **54**

110g rye or wholemeal flour

1 tsp bicarbonate of soda

½ tsp ground cinnamon

75g walnuts (or pecans) roughly chopped

75g firm dried figs, sliced

50g sunflower seeds

pinch of salt

50g honey

200ml buttermilk

FIG & WALNUT CRACKERS

We've used the double-baking method for our crunchy crackers: you cook the dough as a loaf first, then slice and bake the slices until crisp. We know these have to be in the oven for a while but they are really easy to make. Much tastier than most shop-bought crackers, these are great with cheese or with the dips on page 56.

Preheat the oven to 170°C/Fan 150°C/Gas 31/2 and line a small, 450g loaf tin with some baking parchment.

Put the flour, bicarbonate of soda, cinnamon, nuts, figs and sunflower seeds into a bowl. Add a generous pinch of salt, then stir to combine. Drizzle the honey into the buttermilk, then pour the mixture over the dry ingredients and mix to form a batter.

Pour the mixture into the prepared loaf tin and bake in the oven for 35–40 minutes until the loaf is firm, slightly springy and a rich golden-brown colour.

Leave the loaf to cool for as long as you can – the cooler it is, the easier it is to slice. If possible, wrap the loaf and chill it for several hours.

When you are ready for the second bake, preheat the oven to 150°C/Fan 130°C/Gas 2. Slice the loaf as thinly as you can – you should get about 30 slices. Arrange the slices on a couple of baking trays, then put them in the oven and bake until they have taken on more colour and are fairly crisp – this will take 20–30 minutes.

Remove the crackers from the oven and transfer them to a cooling rack. They will continue to crisp up as they cool. Store in an airtight container.

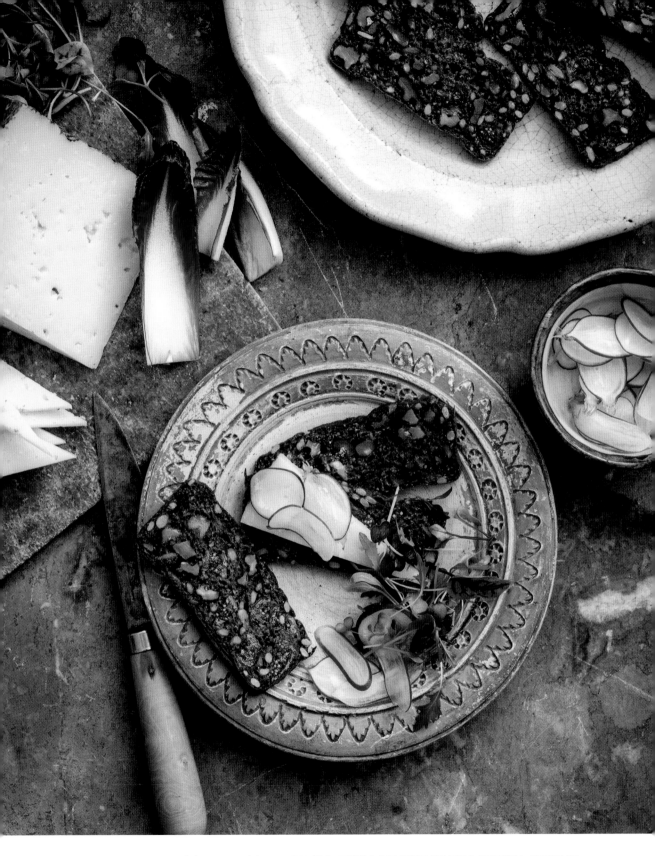

INFO PER CRACKER: PROTEIN (G) 1.5 CARBS (G) 5.5 SUGAR (G) 3 FAT (G) 3 SATURATED FAT (G) 0.5 FIBRE (G) 1 SALT (G) 0.2

Makes: **1 loaf**
(about 12 slices)

 Prep: **15 minutes, plus
rising time**

 Cooking time:
35–45 minutes

 Calories per slice with
serving options/
without: **254/212**

BLACK BREAD WITH SEEDS

250ml strong coffee (hot)

25ml apple cider vinegar

2 tbsp treacle, molasses
   or malt extract

1 tbsp honey

2 tbsp olive oil

300g dark rye flour

200g strong white plain flour

20g cocoa powder

1 heaped tsp salt

7g instant yeast (1 sachet)

50g sunflower seeds

½ tsp of fennel, anise or
   caraway seeds (optional)

TO SERVE (OPTIONAL)

125g cream cheese

2–3 tsp wasabi paste

100g smoked salmon, pulled
   into strips

1 tbsp sushi ginger, finely
   chopped

1 tbsp ponzu

a few microleaves

salt and black pepper

This is a really good flavourful bread. Enjoy it as it is with a bit of butter or turn it into a light meal with cream cheese and smoked salmon. Ponzu has a lovely citrusy flavour which goes beautifully with the salmon, but if you don't have any, use soy sauce and a squeeze of lemon juice instead.

Line a 900g loaf tin with baking parchment. Put the coffee in a jug and add the cider vinegar, treacle, molasses or malt extract, honey and olive oil. Whisk together and set aside while you mix together the dry ingredients.

Put the flours into a mixing bowl with the cocoa and salt. Mix well, then sprinkle in the yeast and whatever seeds you're using and mix again. Make a well in the centre of the flour and gradually work in the wet ingredients until you have a very sticky dough. Knead for a few minutes until the dough is smooth and less sticky – it won't become as elastic as a regular bread dough.

Cover with a damp cloth and leave to stand until the dough has risen. It probably won't quite double in size, but when it has risen to a smooth dome, knock it back and shape it into a loaf. Put it into the loaf tin and leave to rise for a second time.

Preheat the oven to 200°C/Fan 180°C/Gas 6. Bake the bread for 35–45 minutes. Check that the loaf is ready by making sure it sounds hollow when you tap the base, then leave it to cool on a rack. It will keep very well.

One idea for serving – mix the cream cheese with the wasabi paste until smooth and spread it over 4 slices of the bread. Toss the salmon with the ginger and ponzu, then season with salt and pepper. Arrange the salmon over the cream cheese and top with a few microleaves.

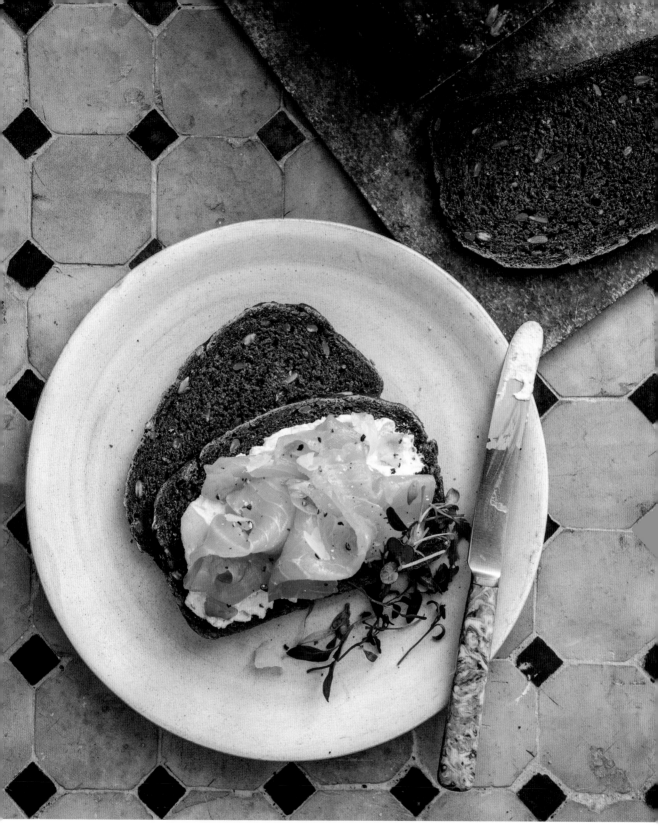

INFO PER SLICE WITH SERVING OPTIONS/WITHOUT: PROTEIN (G) 8/5.5 CARBS (G) 35/34.5 SUGAR (G) 4.5/4 FAT (G) 8/5

SATURATED FAT (G) 2.5/1 FIBRE (G) 5/5 SALT (G) 0.9/0.4

Serves: **4 or more**

 Prep: **10 minutes each**

 Cooking time:
no cooking

 Calories per 30g
Roast red pepper: **37**
Sunblush tomato: **50**

DELICIOUS DIPS

ROAST RED PEPPER DIP

250g roast red peppers
(from a jar or roast your own)

2–3 tsp harissa paste

1 garlic clove, chopped

zest and juice of ½ lemon

½ tsp dried thyme

50g almond butter

100g Greek yoghurt

salt and black pepper

TO SERVE

1 tbsp olive oil

1–2 preserved lemons, finely
chopped

a few parsley or mint leaves

Remove any seeds from the peppers. Put the peppers into a food processor along with 2 teaspoons of the harissa paste, the garlic, lemon zest and juice and the thyme. Add salt and pepper and blitz until smooth. Add the almond butter and process again to combine, then finally add the Greek yoghurt. Taste and stir in the remaining harissa paste if you want the dip to be a bit spicier.

Transfer to a bowl or a container and chill until ready to serve. Give the dip a good stir, then garnish with a drizzle of olive oil, some finely chopped preserved lemon and a sprinkling of parsley or mint.

SUNBLUSH TOMATO & ANCHOVY DIP

30g tin of anchovies and their oil

100g sunblush tomatoes and 1 tbsp
of their oil

2 tbsp tomato purée

1 garlic clove, crushed or grated

zest and juice of ½ lemon

1 tsp chilli powder

1 small bunch of parsley, roughly
chopped

leaves from 2 large basil sprigs

1 tbsp red wine vinegar

25g capers

½ tsp honey (optional)

salt and black pepper

Put all the ingredients, except the honey, into a food processor. Add plenty of black pepper but hold off on the salt to start with. Process everything together, using the pulse function at first until a paste starts to form, pushing the mixture down as necessary. Process until you have a flecked paste – it shouldn't be too smooth.

Taste for seasoning and add a little salt if necessary. You can also adjust the other flavours if you like, adding more chilli or lemon. If you find the dip too sharp or astringent, add the honey and mix to combine.

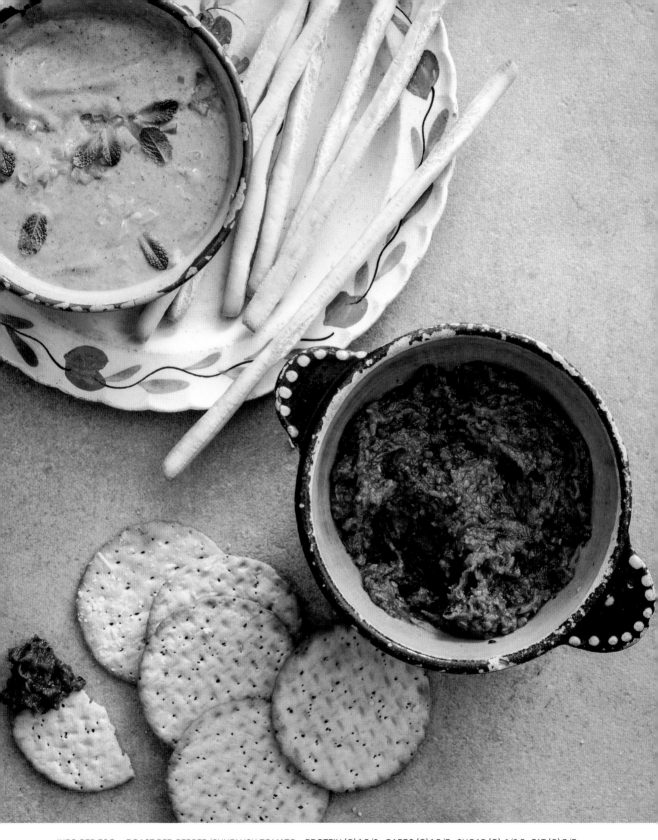

INFO PER 30G — ROAST RED PEPPER/SUNBLUSH TOMATO: PROTEIN (G) 1.5/2 CARBS (G) 1.5/3 SUGAR (G) 1/2.5 FAT (G) 3/3

SATURATED FAT (G) 0.5/0.5 FIBRE (G) 0/1 SALT (G) 0.1/0.9

Serves: **4**

 Prep: **5 minutes**

 Cooking time: **5–10 minutes**

 Calories per serving with toast: **218**

TOMATO & RICOTTA TOAST TOPPER

2 tbsp olive oil

24–36 cherry tomatoes (depending on size)

2 garlic cloves, finely chopped

leaves from a thyme sprig (or ½ tsp dried)

2 tsp white or dark balsamic vinegar

1 tbsp lemon juice

zest of ½ lemon

150g ricotta

a few mint or basil leaves

salt and black pepper

I had a version of this in an Italian motorway restaurant recently and thought it was fab. Good on chunky sourdough, bruschetta-style, or on an ordinary piece of toast when you fancy a snack. You could roast the tomatoes, but this pan-frying method is faster and much more economical on fuel – and it works really well. (Si)

Heat the olive oil in a lidded sauté pan. Add the cherry tomatoes and season them with salt and pepper. Cover the pan and sauté the tomatoes over a medium-low heat for several minutes, shaking the pan at intervals, until they are lightly browned and close to bursting. Add the garlic and thyme and gently stir to coat, then add the balsamic vinegar and lemon juice.

Stir the lemon zest into the ricotta. Spread this over toast and spoon the tomatoes and their dressing over the top. Finish with a few fresh mint or basil leaves and a good crack of black pepper.

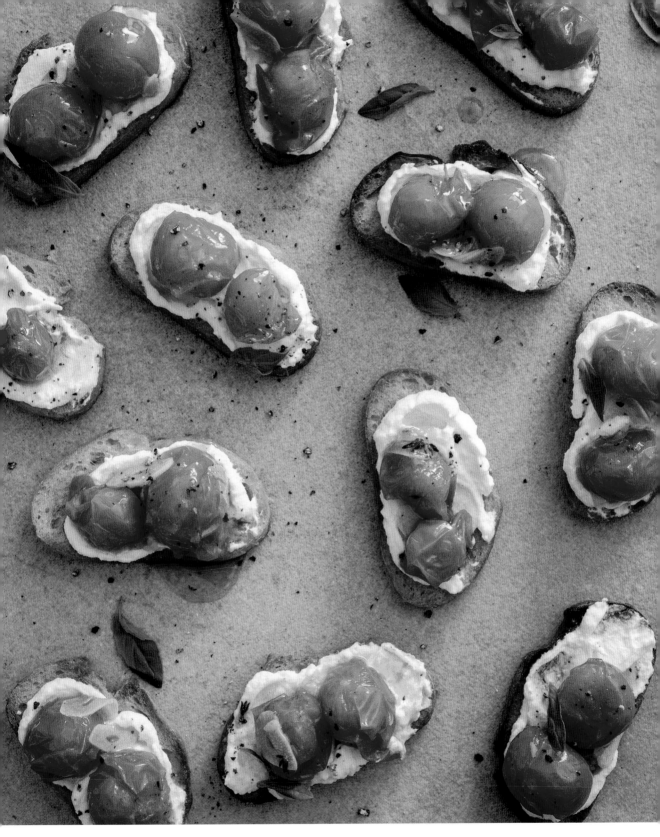

INFO PER SERVING (WITH TOAST): PROTEIN (G) 8.5 CARBS (G) 19.5 SUGAR (G) 4.5 FAT (G) 11 SATURATED FAT (G) 3.5
FIBRE (G) 4 SALT (G) 0.5

Makes: **4**

 Prep: **10–15 minutes, plus standing time**

 Cooking time: **about 30 minutes**

 Calories per flatbread: **412**

FLATBREADS WITH TURMERIC & BLACK PEPPER

150g gram (chickpea) flour

150g strong white or wholemeal plain flour

1 tbsp baking powder

1 tsp ground turmeric

1 tsp cumin seeds

1 tsp ground black peppercorns

1 tsp salt

150ml plain yoghurt

2 tbsp olive oil

1 egg, beaten

olive oil or butter, for cooking and brushing

Gram or chickpea flour is available in supermarkets and makes wonderful flatbreads. We like to mix gram flour half and half with regular flour for the best flavour and texture. These little beauties are just the job with the lentil pâté on page 62 or the dips on page 56, so get baking and give them a go.

Put the flours, baking powder and spices into a bowl with a teaspoon of salt. Whisk to combine and to remove the lumps in the gram flour, then stir in the yoghurt, oil and egg. Stir until you have a fairly stiff dough.

Divide the mixture into 4 pieces and flatten each one out into a teardrop-shaped flatbread. Cover them with a tea towel and leave to stand for at least 20 minutes. You'll find that they won't necessarily have risen, but the dough will be softer and slightly puffy at this stage.

Heat a frying pan or a griddle and rub it with a little olive oil or butter. Cook the flatbreads one at a time until they are cooked through and dappled brown – they will only need 3–4 minutes on each side – then brush with a little oil or butter. Wrap the flatbreads in a tea towel once cooked – this will keep them warm and soft.

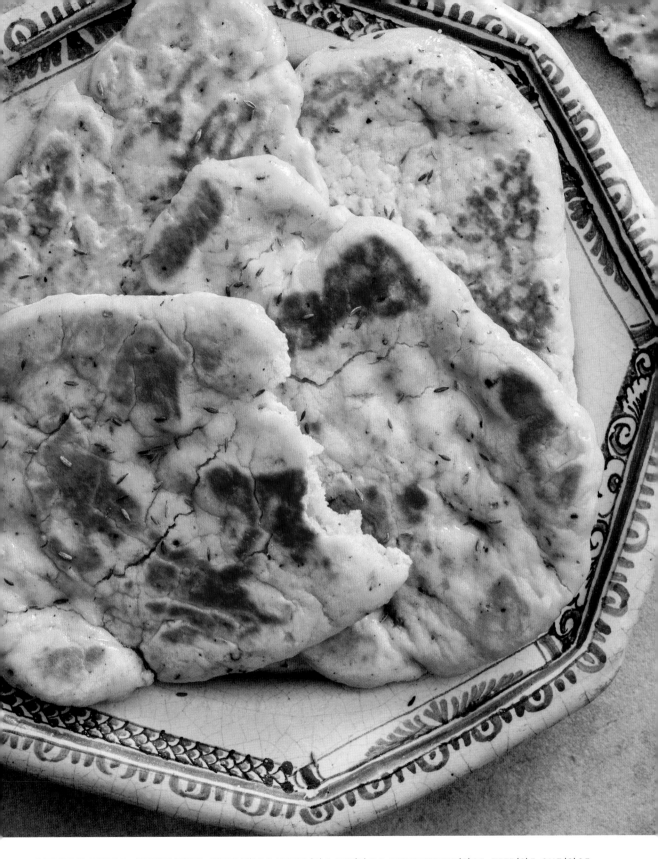

INFO PER FLATBREAD: PROTEIN (G) 17.5 CARBS (G) 52.5 SUGAR (G) 4 FAT (G) 13.5 SATURATED FAT (G) 2.5 FIBRE (G) 5 SALT (G) 2.3

Serves: **4**

Prep: **15 minutes**

Cooking time:
up to 10 minutes

Calories per 50g: **85**

LENTIL & ALMOND PÂTÉ

1 tbsp olive oil

1 small onion, very finely chopped

3 garlic cloves, very finely chopped

250g cooked brown or green lentils

25g ground almonds

½ tsp ground turmeric

½ tsp ground cinnamon

½ tsp chilli powder (optional)

1 tsp dried mint

zest of 1 lemon

1 tbsp lemon juice

leaves from a small bunch of parsley, finely chopped, plus extra to serve

1 tbsp za'atar, to serve

salt and black pepper

An excellent vegetarian pâté, this has a lovely savoury flavour, with a hint of sweetness from the almonds and cinnamon. The almonds also help to thicken the mixture to a nice spreadable texture. Try it with toast or the flatbreads on page 60 and you're in for a treat.

Heat the olive oil in a small frying pan, add the onion and sauté until soft and translucent. Add 2 of the garlic cloves and fry for another couple of minutes, then transfer everything to a food processor.

Process the onion for a few moments, then add all the remaining ingredients, including the rest of the garlic. Season with plenty of salt and pepper and process until you have a thick paste. You can make the mixture as smooth as you like but we prefer to keep it with a bit of texture.

Scoop the mixture into a container and chill it in the fridge. Sprinkle with some za'atar and a little more parsley and serve with hot buttered toast or warm flatbreads.

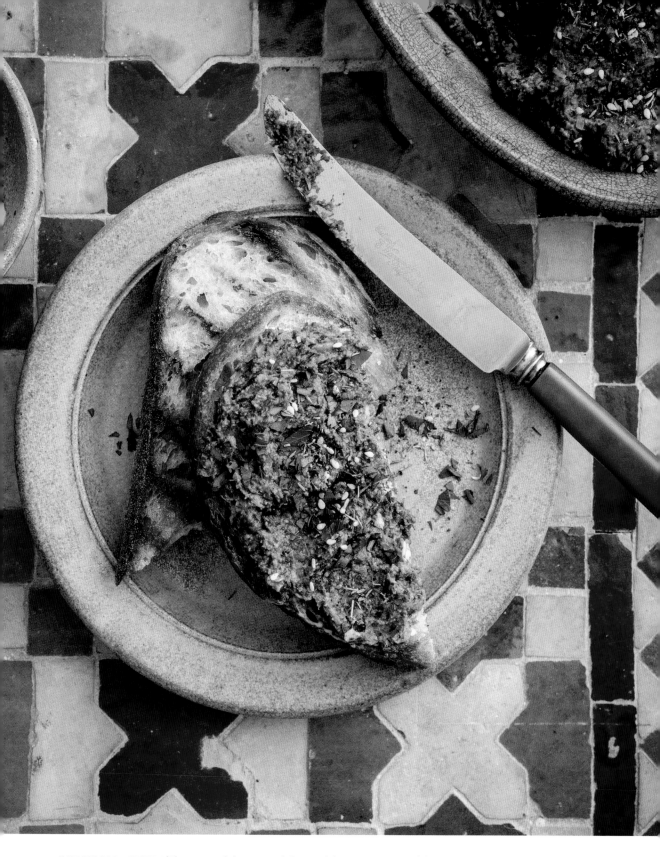

INFO PER 50G: PROTEIN (G) 4   CARBS (G) 7   SUGAR (G) 1   FAT (G) 4   SATURATED FAT (G) 0.5   FIBRE (G) 2.5   SALT (G) TRACE

Serves: **4**

 Prep: **10 minutes**

 Cooking time:
no cooking

 Calories per serving:
142

1 avocado
juice of ½ lime
4 medium tomatoes, sliced
    into rounds
300g silken tofu, sliced and
    chilled

DRESSING
2 tbsp dark soy sauce
5g root ginger, grated
1 tsp honey
juice of ½ lime

TO GARNISH
2 spring onions, cut into 4cm
    lengths and shredded
1 tsp sesame oil
a few basil leaves, shredded
salt

TOFU WITH TOMATO & AVOCADO

For the tofu lovers out there, this is a vegan version of the famous Italian tricolore salad – mozzarella, avocado and tomato. It's super-refreshing when the tofu is well chilled, but the avocado and tomatoes have a much better flavour at room temperature, so this is best assembled just before serving. An attractive little snack whether you're vegan or not.

First, prepare the spring onion garnish. Cut the spring onions into pieces about 4cm long and shred them. Season with salt and cover them with iced water – this will help them to curl up nicely.

Mix all the dressing ingredients together and leave to stand for a few minutes.

Peel and slice the avocado and toss it in the lime juice. Arrange the avocado slices, tomatoes and tofu slices on a large plate and drizzle over the dressing, followed by the sesame oil. Drain the spring onions and sprinkle them over the top with the basil leaves. Best served straight away.

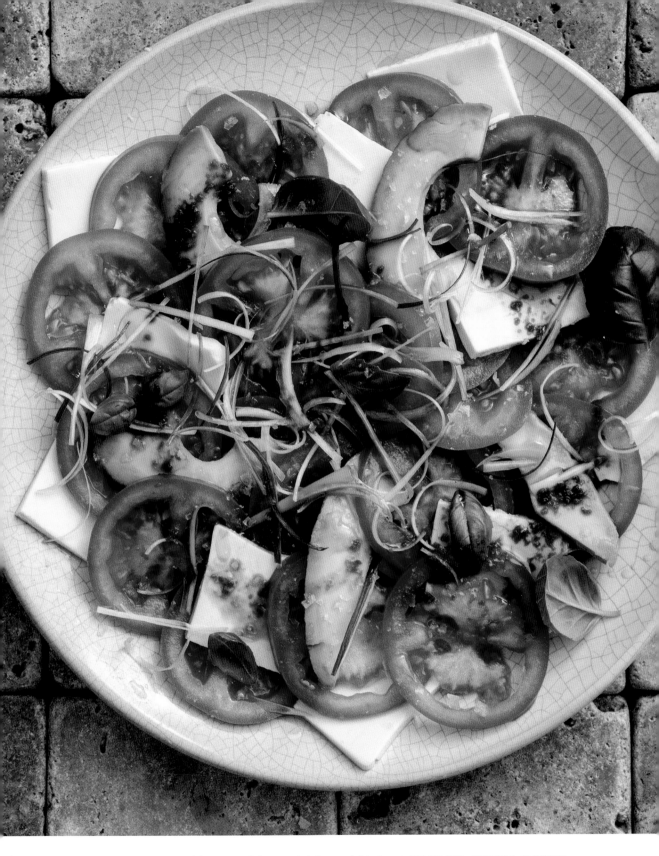

INFO PER SERVING: PROTEIN (G) 6 CARBS (G) 7 SUGAR (G) 6 FAT (G) 9 SATURATED FAT (G) 2 FIBRE (G) 2 SALT (G) 1.1

Makes: **20**

 Prep: **15 minutes**, plus standing time

 Cooking time: **20–30 minutes**

 Calories per fritter fried/baked: **44/32**

VEGETABLE FRITTERS

250g cabbage, finely shredded

150g carrot, cut into matchsticks or coarsely grated

75g radishes, cut into fine matchsticks

3 spring onions, finely chopped

2 tbsp coriander stems, finely chopped

salt and black pepper

BATTER

85g gram (chickpea) flour

15g cornflour

½ tsp ground turmeric

½ tsp cayenne powder

1 tsp ground cumin

1 tsp mustard seeds

1 tsp baking powder

TO OVEN BAKE

olive oil, for greasing

2 tsp coconut oil

TO FRY

3–4 tbsp olive or vegetable oil

TO SERVE

lemon or lime wedges

a sprinkling of cayenne

We do like a fritter and these are a cross between a rösti and a bhaji. The gram flour batter is just enough to make a nice coating, so the vegetables are the hero here and they crisp up like little nests. You can fry the fritters or bake them – up to you. We find that they crisp up better when fried, but cooking them in the oven is simpler and uses less oil. See how you feel on the day. Nice with something like a bowl of raita.

Put the prepared cabbage, carrot and radishes into a colander and sprinkle them with half a teaspoon of salt. Mix thoroughly, then leave to stand for half an hour. Transfer the veg to a tea towel and gently squeeze out any excess liquid.

For the batter, put the gram flour, cornflour, spices and baking powder into a bowl and add a generous amount of salt and black pepper. Whisk in 100ml of water to make a fairly thick batter. Add the salted and squeezed vegetables, the spring onions and coriander stems and mix thoroughly.

To oven bake the fritters, preheat the oven to 200°C/Fan 180°C/Gas 6 and rub a couple of baking trays with oil. Spoon heaped tablespoons of the mixture on to the baking trays, spacing them out well, then flatten them a little. The mixture should make about 20. Melt 2 teaspoons of coconut oil and brush a few drops over each fritter, then bake for about 20 minutes, flipping them halfway through.

To fry, heat a tablespoon of oil in a large frying pan. Drop heaped tablespoons of the mixture on to the frying pan and flatten them slightly, then cook over a high heat until they are crisp underneath and holding together. Flip and repeat until crisp on both sides. Drain on kitchen paper and repeat, adding more oil as necessary, until you have used up all the fritter mixture.

Serve with a squeeze of lemon or lime and a sprinkling of extra cayenne for more heat.

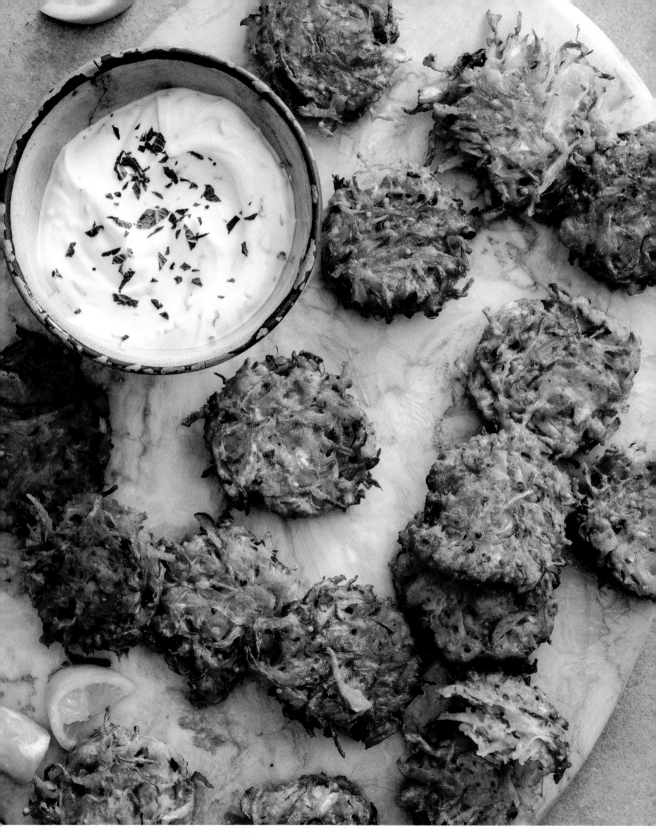

INFO PER FRITTER – FRIED/BAKED: PROTEIN (G) 1.5/1.5   CARBS (G) 4/4   SUGAR (G) 1/1   FAT (G) 2/1   SATURATED FAT (G) 0.5/0.5

FIBRE (G) 1/1   SALT (G) TRACE/TRACE

Makes: **16**

 Prep: **10 minutes**

 Cooking time:
no cooking

 Calories per bomb: **103**

100g tahini

75g honey

zest of ½ orange

50g rolled oats

50g flaked almonds

25g cacao or cocoa powder

½ tsp ground cinnamon

2 tbsp sesame or chia seeds

pinch of salt

COATING

cocoa powder or sesame
    seeds

CHOCOLATE & TAHINI ENERGY BOMBS

Pop some of these in your fridge for those moments when you need a bit of an energy boost. Tahini is really popular in Middle Eastern cooking and is just as good in sweet dishes as in savoury. It marries perfectly with the chocolate and orange in this recipe.

Put the tahini and honey into a bowl and stir in the orange zest. Put the rolled oats and flaked almonds into a small food processor and pulse until they're a bit more broken up, but not ground to a powder.

Add the oat and nut mixture to the tahini and honey along with the cocoa powder, cinnamon and sesame or chia seeds. Add a pinch of salt and mix thoroughly – the mixture will eventually clump together.

Divide the mixture into 16 balls and roll each one in cocoa powder or some sesame seeds to coat. Chill in the fridge.

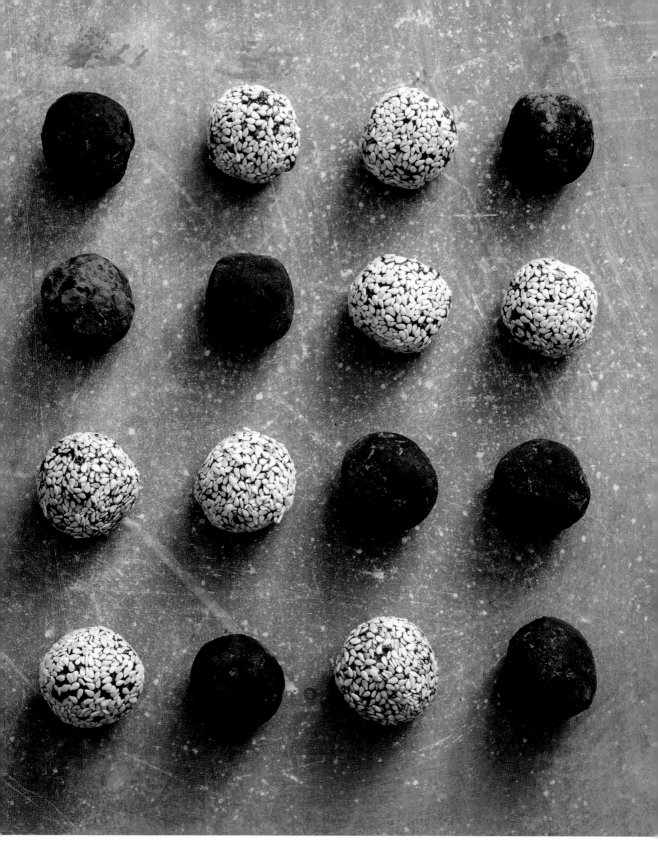

INFO PER BOMB: PROTEIN (G) 3   CARBS (G) 6   SUGAR (G) 3.5   FAT (G) 7   SATURATED FAT (G) 1   FIBRE (G) 1.5   SALT (G) 0.1

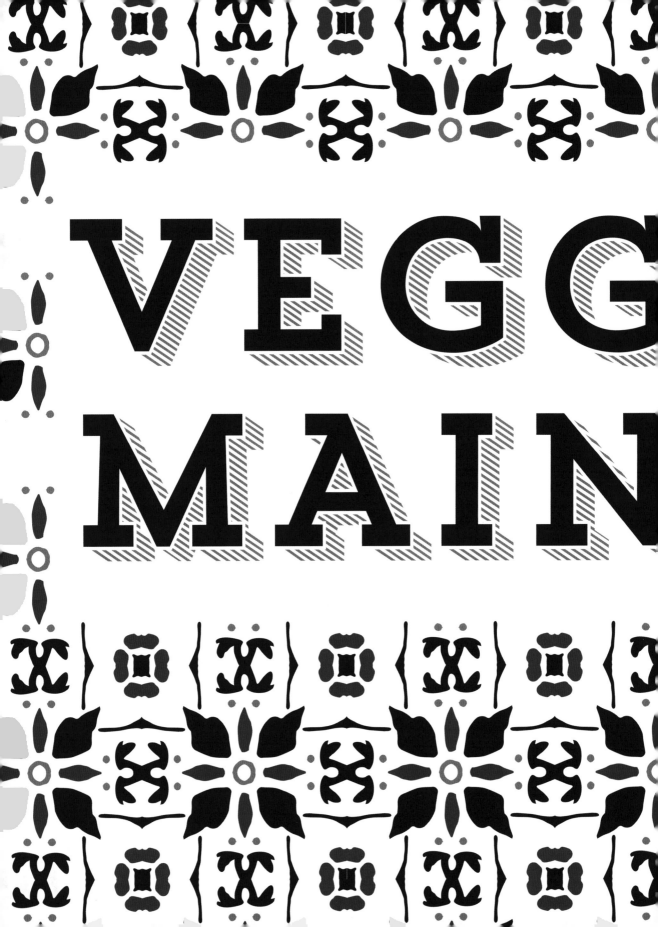

VEGG
MAIN

IES

CHICKPEA & BROAD BEAN FALAFEL

CAULIFLOWER RICE RISOTTO

EGYPTIAN BEAN STEW

GREEK GIANT BEANS

PERFECT PESTOS

AUBERGINES WITH SOBA NOODLES

SQUASH & COURGETTE GRATIN

SPINACH & HALLOUMI CURRY

PERSIAN HERB OMELETTE

PASTA WITH CHILLI & LENTILS

SQUASH & QUINOA RISOTTO

Serves: **4**

 Prep: **20 minutes, plus chilling time**

 Cooking time: **about 30 minutes**

 Calories per serving with pitta/without: **574/390**

CHICKPEA & BROAD BEAN FALAFEL

25g gram (chickpea) flour
    or plain flour
300g frozen broad beans
400g can of chickpeas,
    drained
1 small onion, finely chopped
2 garlic cloves, finely chopped
10g parsley, finely chopped
zest of ½ lemon
1 tsp dried mint
1 tsp ground cumin
½ tsp ground cinnamon
1 tsp baking powder
olive oil, for frying
salt and black pepper

TAHINI SAUCE
100g tahini, well mixed
1 tsp honey
1 garlic clove, finely chopped
juice of ½ lemon
125ml warm water

TO SERVE
pitta breads
lemon wedges
cucumber slices
pickled red cabbage
    (optional)

Falafels are often made just with chickpeas but we think a mix of chickpeas and broad beans is even better and produces a tastier result. Toasting the gram flour, if using, might seem a faff but is well worth it for the improvement in flavour. These tasty morsels are easy to prepare with the help of a food processor and they slip down very nicely with the tahini sauce.

If using gram (chickpea) flour, sprinkle it into a dry frying pan and toast, stirring regularly, until it smells rich and nutty. This is just to cook out the raw flavour.

Next peel the broad beans. The easiest way to do this is to pour a kettle of freshly boiled water over them and leave them to stand for a minute. You will find that the skins then slip off very easily.

Put the broad beans into a food processor with all the remaining falafel ingredients, except the olive oil, and season with salt and black pepper. Pulse until everything has broken down a little. Allow the mixture at the bottom of the food processor to get quite smooth, then stir and pulse again. You want to keep some texture, so don't overdo the processing.

Scoop the mixture into a bowl or container and leave to chill in the fridge for half an hour to firm up. Remove from the fridge and divide into 16 small patties. Put the patties back in the fridge until you are ready to fry them.

While the falafel mixture is chilling, make the tahini sauce. Put all the ingredients, except the warm water, in a small food processor and pulse until well mixed. Add enough of the water to make a sauce with the consistency of double cream.

Cover the base of a frying pan with olive oil. When it's hot, fry the falafel, a few at a time, over a medium heat. They will take 3–4 minutes on each side. Place each batch on kitchen paper to drain.

Check the consistency of the sauce just before serving and add a little more warm water and/or lemon juice if it needs it. Serve the falafel in warm pitta breads with the tahini sauce, lemon wedges, cucumber and perhaps some pickled red cabbage.

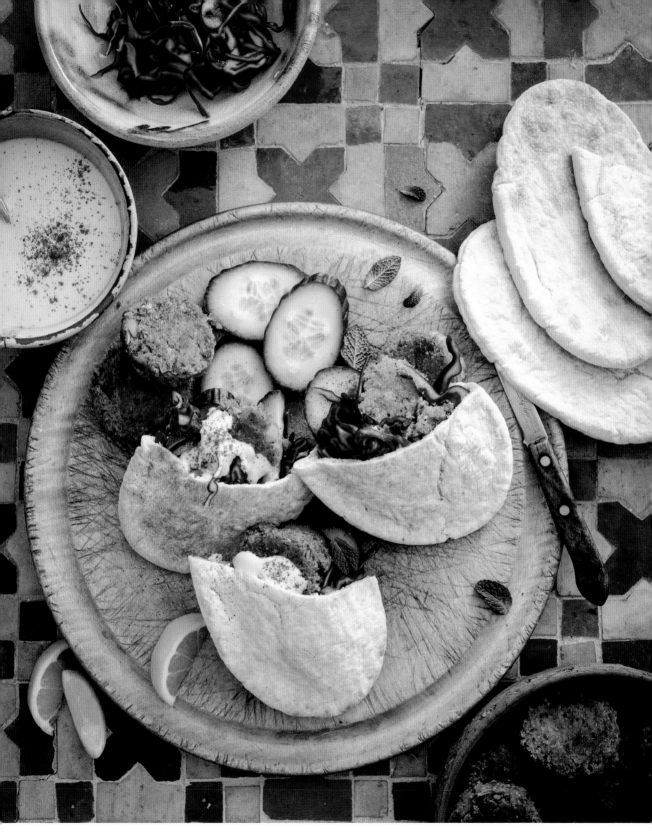

INFO PER SERVING WITH PITTA/WITHOUT: PROTEIN (G) 23/16   CARBS (G) 59/22   SUGAR (G) 6/4   FAT (G) 24/23   SATURATED FAT (G) 3/3

FIBRE (G) 15/13   SALT (G) 1/0.3

CAULIFLOWER RICE RISOTTO

 Serves: **4**

 Prep: **15 minutes**

 Cooking time:
about 25 minutes

 Calories per serving:
336

3 tbsp olive oil

1 cauliflower (500–600g),
   broken into florets

1 bunch of asparagus

2 garlic cloves, finely chopped

1 lime

15g butter

1 onion, finely chopped

1 medium courgette, finely
   diced

100g peas (frozen are fine and
   it's OK to use from frozen)

a few lemon thyme leaves

100ml white wine

125g cream cheese

25g vegetarian Parmesan-
   style cheese, grated, plus
   extra to serve

salt and black pepper

Making a risotto with cauliflower instead of rice is a great trick for cutting calories while still producing a pleasing and comforting dish. We wanted to prevent the cauliflower going soggy and found that the combination of boiling and steaming in the final stage gave just the right result. If you fancy, you could add in some spinach or rocket at the end to wilt in the heat before serving.

Heat a tablespoon of the oil in a large sauté pan. When it's hot, add the cauliflower florets and sear them until lightly browned in patches. Transfer them to a food processor and process until they resemble fine breadcrumbs. It's best to do this in a few batches so you don't end up with an uneven texture.

Prepare the asparagus. Snap off the woody ends and save them for stock, then cut off the tips and set them aside. Finely slice the remainder of the stems into rounds. Heat another tablespoon of oil in the pan. Sauté the asparagus rounds until just cooked through – al dente – then add one of the garlic cloves and a rasp of lime zest. Season with salt and pepper. Stir to combine and cook the garlic for a minute, then remove everything from the pan and set aside.

Heat the remainder of the olive oil with the butter in the sauté pan. Add the onion and cook until soft and translucent, then add the asparagus stem rounds, the courgette, peas and cauliflower. Sauté for a minute or so until everything is well coated in the oil and butter, then stir in the remaining garlic and the lemon thyme. Season with salt and pepper.

Pour in the wine and bring to the boil. Cook, stirring, for a few minutes, until most of the wine has evaporated, then add 150ml of water. Bring to the boil again and simmer, uncovered, for several minutes until most of the water has evaporated, then cover and leave over a low heat to steam gently for 5 minutes. After this, the cauliflower should be completely cooked through.

Stir in the cream cheese with a little more water to loosen it, then beat in the grated cheese. The texture should be creamy and not too dry. Add more lime zest and a squeeze of lime juice to the cauliflower, then lay the asparagus tips on top. Cover the pan and leave for a minute or so off the heat just to warm through the asparagus tips, then serve with more grated cheese if you like.

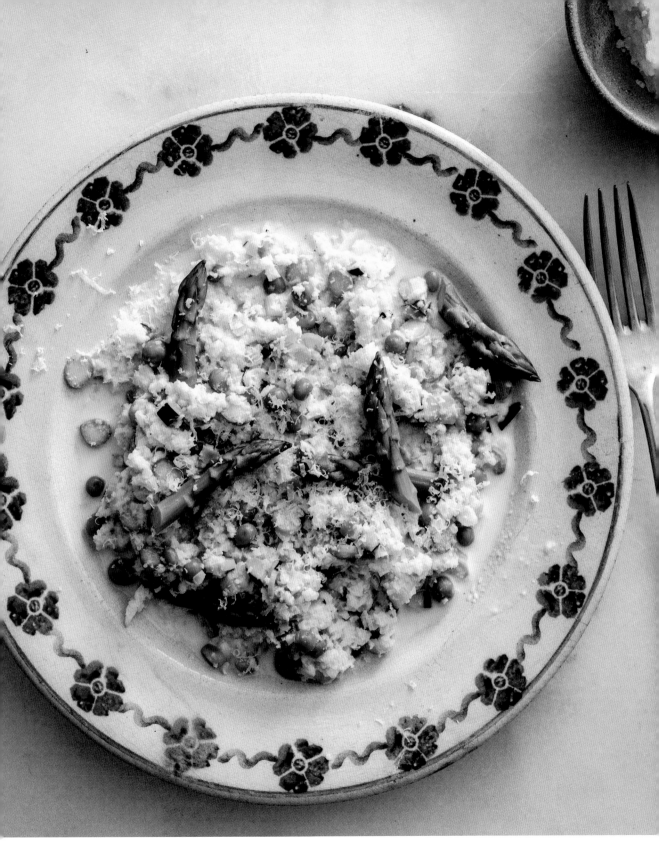

INFO PER SERVING: PROTEIN (G) 12.5   CARBS (G) 15   SUGAR (G) 10   FAT (G) 21.5   SATURATED FAT (G) 9   FIBRE (G) 7   SALT (G) 0.5

Serves: **4**

 Prep: **10 minutes**

Cooking time:
about 15 minutes

 Calories per serving
(without pitta): **247**

EGYPTIAN BEAN STEW

2 tbsp olive oil

1 red onion, finely sliced

3 garlic cloves, finely chopped

1 tsp ground cumin

½ tsp ground cinnamon

zest and juice of 1 lemon

2 x 400g cans of whole fava beans

2 tbsp tahini

salt and black pepper

TO SERVE

1 large tomato, finely diced

small bunch of parsley, finely chopped

2 green chillies, finely sliced

pitta bread (optional)

This is our version of the dish known as ful medames which is much loved throughout the Middle East, but is believed to have originated in Egypt. It's eaten at any time of day and can be topped with almost anything you fancy, including fried eggs. The classic recipe involves soaking and cooking dried beans but using canned beans makes things much quicker and easier. If you can't find fava beans you could use butter beans instead.

Heat the olive oil in a large sauté pan or a flameproof casserole dish. Add the red onion and cook over a medium heat until lightly browned. Add the garlic, cumin, cinnamon and lemon zest, then stir in the beans along with 400ml of water. Season with salt and black pepper. Bring to the boil, then turn down the heat and leave to simmer for about 5 minutes.

Mash some of the beans to create a creamy texture – do this with a potato masher straight in the pan or crush some against the side of the pan with a wooden spoon. Stir in the tahini and half the lemon juice. Taste and adjust the seasoning and add more tahini and lemon juice as necessary.

Season the tomato with salt and pepper and spoon it on top of the beans with the parsley and chillies. Serve with warm pitta bread.

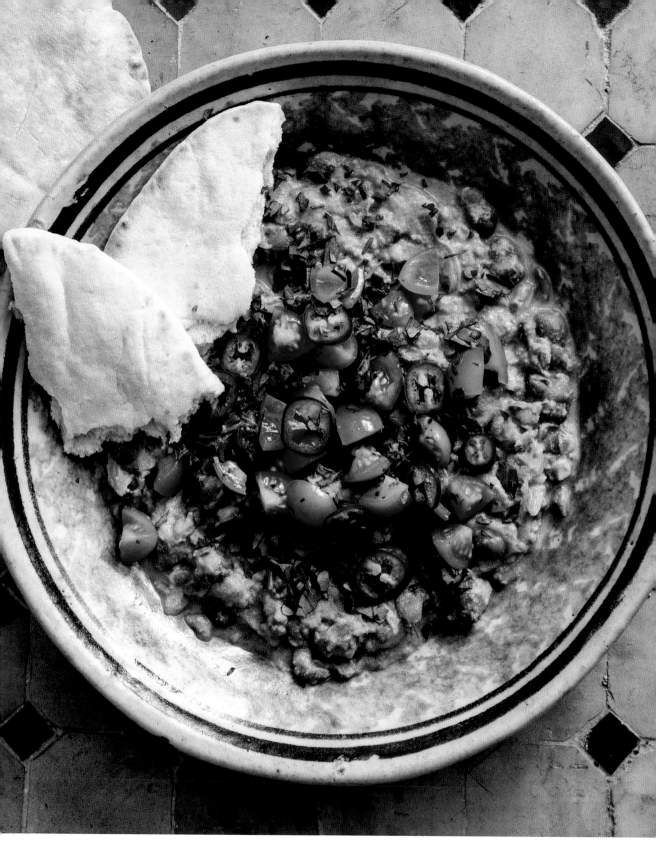

INFO PER SERVING: PROTEIN (G) 13   CARBS (G) 19   SUGAR (G) 4   FAT (G) 11   SATURATED FAT (G) 1.5   FIBRE (G) 11   SALT (G) 0.9

Serves: **4**

Prep: **10 minutes**

Cooking time:
about 50 minutes

Calories per serving:
350

2 tbsp olive oil

1 onion, finely diced

1 celery stick, finely diced

½ fennel bulb, finely diced

1 large carrot, finely diced

4 garlic cloves, finely chopped

small bunch of parsley

2 bay leaves

1 tsp dried oregano

½ tsp ground cinnamon

2 x 400g cans of butter beans,
   drained

400g can of tomatoes

250ml vegetable or chicken
   stock

1–2 tsp red wine vinegar

200g vegetarian feta, cubed

salt and black pepper

GREEK GIANT BEANS

Known as gigantes plaki, these beans feature on many a taverna menu all over Greece. They're great served hot as a warming bean stew or at room temperature as part of a veggie banquet. Filling, nourishing and healthy, these make a bowlful of goodness.

Heat the olive oil in a large flameproof casserole dish or a saucepan, then add the onion, celery, fennel and carrot. Sauté over a medium heat for 5 minutes, then add 50ml of water, cover the pan and cook gently for about 10 minutes until the vegetables are tender. Add the garlic and cook for another couple of minutes.

Separate the parsley stems from the leaves and set the leaves aside. Finely chop the stems and add them to the pan with the bay leaves and oregano. Sprinkle in the cinnamon, followed by the beans and tomatoes. Rinse out the tomato can with the stock and add this to the pan, then stir to combine. Season with salt and pepper.

Bring to the boil, then turn the heat down to a simmer and leave to cook, partially covered, for about 30 minutes, until the sauce has reduced around the beans and everything is tender. Add a teaspoon of red wine vinegar, then taste and add another teaspoonful if you think it necessary.

Push the cubes of feta into the beans, then leave to simmer for a few more minutes until the feta is soft and creamy. Roughly chop the parsley leaves and sprinkle them over the beans before serving.

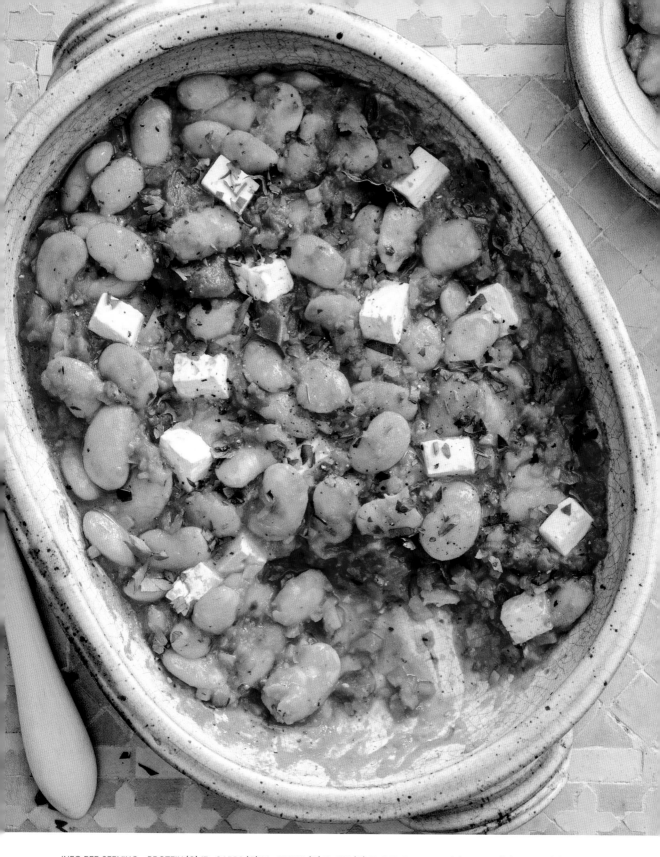

INFO PER SERVING: PROTEIN (G) 17   CARBS (G) 26   SUGAR (G) 11   FAT (G) 17   SATURATED FAT (G) 8   FIBRE (G) 12   SALT (G) 1.4

Serves: **4**

Prep: **10 minutes each**

Cooking time:
no cooking

Calories per tbsp:
Almond & lemon: **66**
Rocket & walnut: **55**

PERFECT PESTOS

ALMOND & LEMON PESTO

75g whole or flaked almonds

25g parsley

a few basil leaves

1 garlic clove, sliced

zest of 2 lemons

juice of 1 lemon

3 tbsp olive oil

½ tsp chilli flakes

salt and black pepper

Put the almonds, parsley, basil, garlic and lemon zest into a food processor and season with salt and pepper. Process in short bursts to start with, pushing the leaves down a couple of times until they have combined with the almonds. At this point, add the lemon juice and drizzle in the olive oil while the motor is running. Continue to push everything down at intervals so it processes evenly.

When everything has been finely chopped and forms a paste, add the chilli flakes. Process one more time, then transfer the pesto to a container and store in the fridge. No cheese in this one so a good vegan option, although you could add cheese at the table if you like.

Both these pestos are great with pasta, gnocchi or whatever you fancy.

ROCKET & WALNUT PESTO

50g rocket

25g baby leaf spinach

25g watercress

a few basil leaves

50g walnuts or pecans, lightly toasted

25g vegetarian Parmesan-style
   cheese, coarsely grated

zest of 1 lemon

1 garlic clove, roughly chopped

50ml olive oil

salt and black pepper

Put all the leaves, the nuts, cheese, lemon zest and garlic into a food processor and season with salt and black pepper. Process with the pulse function to start with, pushing the leaves down until they have combined with the other ingredients. When everything has broken down into a very coarse paste, add the olive oil while the motor is running and process, stopping every so often to push everything down from the sides. You will end up with a deep-green flecked, textured sauce. Transfer to a container and store in the fridge until needed.

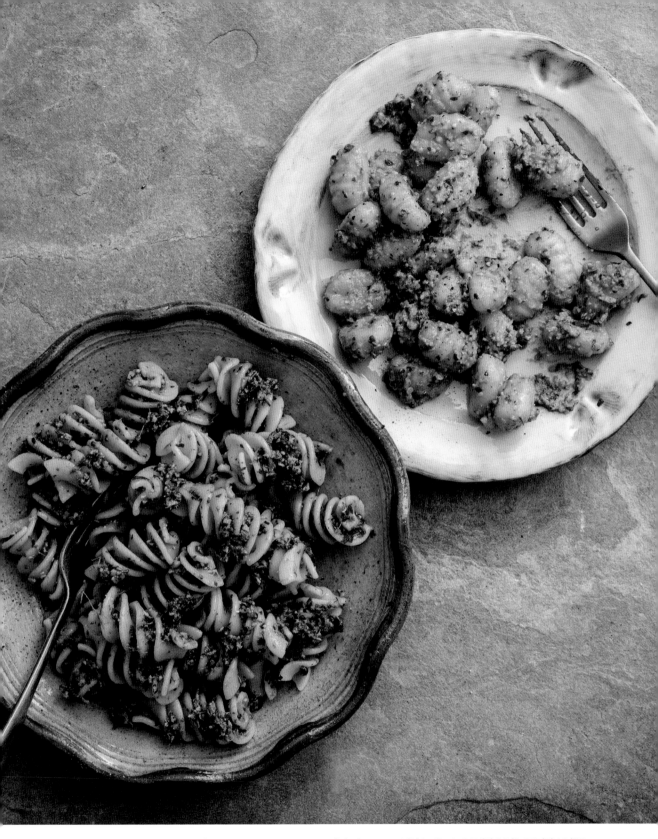

INFO PER TBSP – ALMOND & LEMON/ROCKET & WALNUT: PROTEIN (G) 2/1.5 CARBS (G) 0.5/0 SUGAR (G) 0.5/0 FAT (G) 6.5/5.5
SATURATED FAT (G) 0.5/1 FIBRE (G) 0/0.5 SALT (G) TRACE/TRACE

Serves: **4**

 Prep: **15 minutes**

 Cooking time:
about 20 minutes

 Calories per serving:
300

AUBERGINES WITH SOBA NOODLES

2 large aubergines or same
   weight in baby aubergines
   (600–700g)
5g root ginger, cut into
   matchsticks
3 garlic cloves, very finely
   chopped
salt and black pepper

DRESSING
2 tbsp peanut butter
   (smooth or crunchy)
3 tbsp dark soy sauce
1 tbsp mirin
2 tsp rice vinegar
1 tsp crushed chillies
½ tsp honey

TO SERVE
200g soba noodles
1 tsp sesame oil
100g baby spinach
2 spring onions, finely sliced
1 tsp sesame seeds

This is lovely dish to make if you have any of those little baby aubergines, but it tastes great with any kind. If you're not a fan of peanut butter you could use miso in the dressing instead.

First prepare the aubergines. If using large aubergines, cut them into thick strips. If using baby aubergines, cut them in half lengthways. Place them in a steamer basket and sprinkle over the ginger and garlic, then season with salt and pepper. Set the steamer over a pan of simmering water and steam the aubergines for up to about 15 minutes, until very tender.

Whisk together all the ingredients for the dressing, adding a little water to thin it to a consistency you like, then taste for seasoning and sweetness. Add salt, pepper and a little more honey, if necessary, to get the flavour you want.

Cook the noodles according to the packet instructions and drain them well. Transfer them to a wok or a sauté pan and add the sesame oil, half the dressing and the spinach. Place over a very low heat until the spinach has wilted, then toss gently.

Divide the noodles and spinach between 4 bowls, then top with the aubergines. Pour over the remaining dressing, then top with the spring onions and sesame seeds.

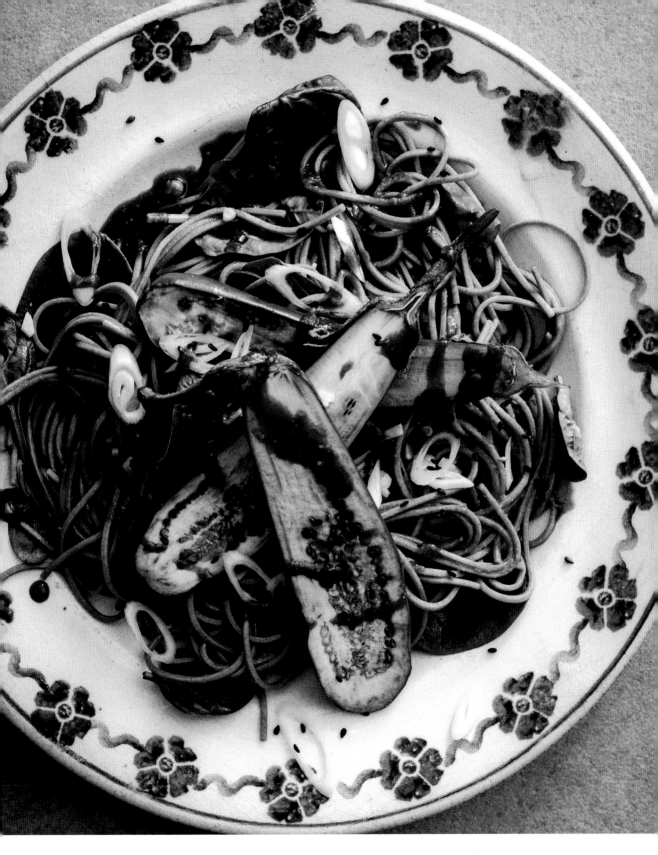

INFO PER SERVING: PROTEIN (G) 12.5 CARBS (G) 42 SUGAR (G) 8 FAT (G) 7.5 SATURATED FAT (G) 1.5 FIBRE (G) 7 SALT (G) 1.7

Serves: **4**

 Prep: **15 minutes**

 Cooking time:
about 45 minutes

 Calories per serving:
273

SQUASH & COURGETTE GRATIN

1 tbsp olive oil

400g butternut squash or similar, peeled and thinly sliced

3 garlic cloves, finely sliced

1 tsp dried thyme or 1 tbsp fresh thyme leaves

25g vegetarian Parmesan-style cheese, finely grated

2 tsp plain flour

150ml single cream

400g courgettes, thinly sliced

a few basil leaves

1 x 125g ball of vegetarian mozzarella, pulled apart

salt and black pepper

An excellent dish whether you're vegetarian or not. If you eat fish, a small can of anchovies gives a great boost of flavour here. Just dice the anchovies and add them with the garlic and thyme.

Preheat the oven to 200°C/Fan 180°C/Gas 6.

Rub a teaspoon of the olive oil over a gratin dish – our dish had a capacity of about 1.5 litres. Arrange half the squash in the base, then season with salt and pepper. Add a few slivers of garlic, some thyme and a sprinkling of grated cheese. Put the plain flour in a small bowl and gradually work in the cream – the flour will help stop the cream from splitting in the oven. Drizzle 2 tablespoons of this mixture over the squash.

Arrange half the courgette slices over the butternut squash, then repeat with more of the seasonings and cream. Repeat the layers with the rest of the butternut squash and courgette, finishing with any remaining seasoning and cream – keep back a little grated cheese to sprinkle over the top later. Dot over a few basil leaves and drizzle over the remaining olive oil.

Cover the dish with foil and bake in the preheated oven for 20 minutes. Check at this point to see if the vegetables are knife tender and cook for a further 5 minutes if necessary. Remove the foil and add the last of the grated cheese and the mozzarella. Bake for a further 15–20 minutes until the gratin is bubbling and lightly browned.

Remove from the oven and leave to rest for at least 5 minutes before serving.

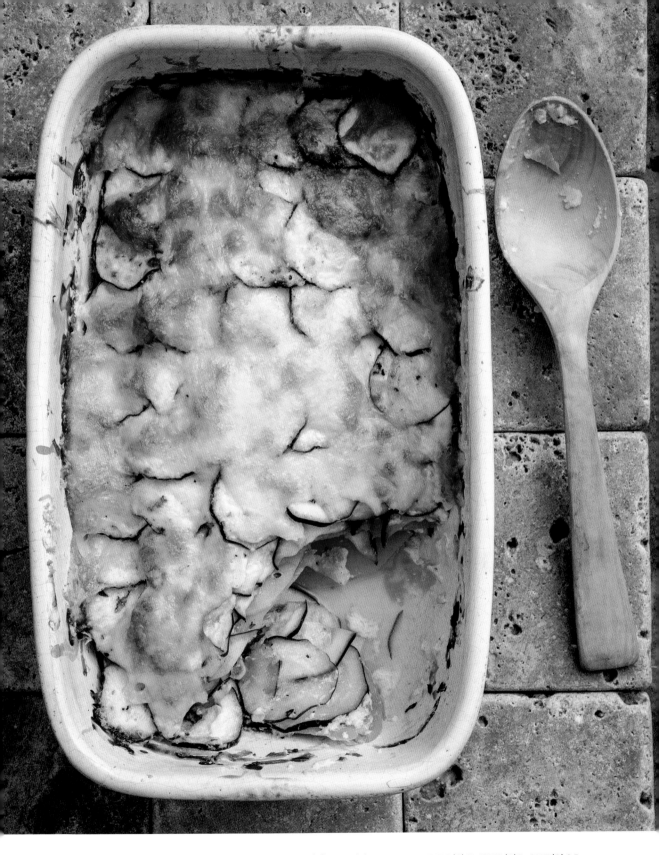

INFO PER SERVING: PROTEIN (G) 12   CARBS (G) 12   SUGAR (G) 7   FAT (G) 19   SATURATED FAT (G) 11   FIBRE (G) 3   SALT (G) 0.5

Serves: **4**

 Prep: **15 minutes**

 Cooking time:
about 30 minutes

 Calories per serving:
438

SPINACH & HALLOUMI CURRY

1 tbsp olive oil

1 tsp cumin seeds

1 large onion, sliced

15g root ginger, grated

4 garlic cloves, grated

1 tbsp medium curry powder

400g can of chopped
    tomatoes

750g frozen whole leaf
    spinach, defrosted

400g can of chickpeas,
    drained

small bunch of coriander,
    finely chopped

squeeze of lemon juice

salt and black pepper

HALLOUMI

1 tbsp olive oil

250g block of vegetarian
    halloumi, cut into large dice

1 tsp dried mint

½ tsp turmeric or curry powder

This curry would normally be made with paneer, but we thought we'd try it with halloumi which has a similar texture and is available in most supermarkets. Made with frozen spinach and canned tomatoes and chickpeas, this is a great store-cupboard dish and is full of flavour and goodness. A perfect weeknight supper.

Heat the olive oil in a large sauté pan or a flameproof casserole dish. Add the cumin seeds and let them sizzle for a few moments, then add the onion. Cook over a medium heat until the onion has taken on some colour and started to soften, then add the ginger, garlic and curry powder.

Cook for another couple of minutes, stirring constantly, then add the tomatoes. Add the spinach and its liquid, along with the chickpeas and most of the coriander. Stir to combine with the spices and season with salt and pepper.

Bring to the boil, then partially cover the pan and turn down the heat. Leave to simmer for 10 minutes.

Meanwhile, cook the halloumi. Heat the olive oil in a large frying pan and when it's hot, add the halloumi. Sear the halloumi on at least a couple of sides and sprinkle with the mint and turmeric or curry powder. Add the halloumi to the pan with the spinach and tomatoes, then simmer for a further 5 minutes, uncovered. Finish with the reserved coriander and a squeeze of lemon juice. Nice served with brown basmati rice.

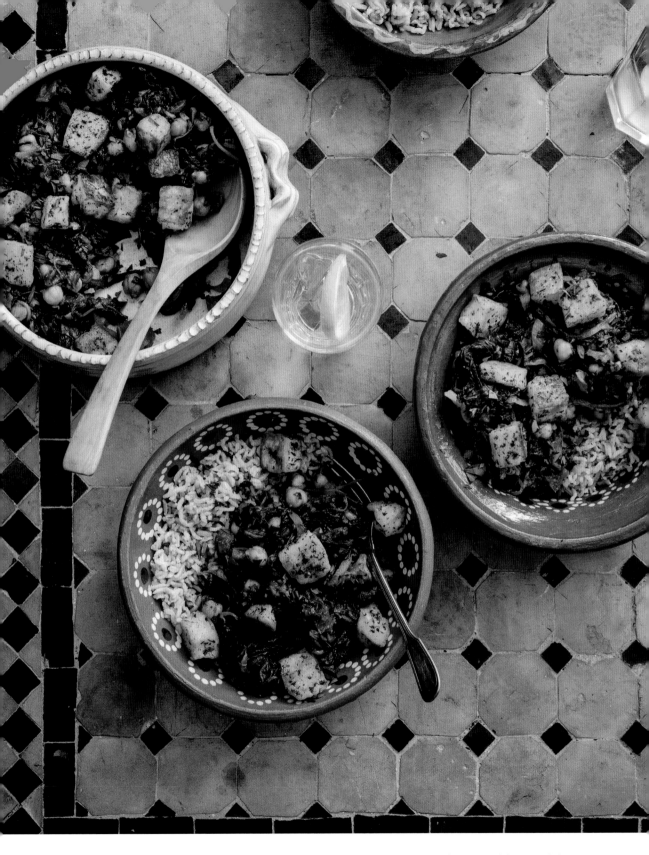

INFO PER SERVING: PROTEIN (G) 27 CARBS (G) 22 SUGAR (G) 11 FAT (G) 24 SATURATED FAT (G) 11.5 FIBRE (G) 12 SALT (G) 2.6

Serves: **4**

 Prep: **15 minutes**

 Cooking time:
about 15 minutes

 Calories per serving:
291

PERSIAN HERB OMELETTE

150g salad potatoes
(unpeeled), finely diced

2 tbsp olive oil

1 onion, finely chopped

75g herbs (any combination of
coriander, parsley, mint, dill,
chervil), roughly chopped

3 garlic cloves, finely chopped

6 eggs

½ tsp ground turmeric

¼ tsp ground cinnamon

1 tbsp barberries

1 tbsp flaked almonds

salt and black pepper

TO SERVE

300g tomatoes, roughly
chopped or sliced

zest and juice of ½ lemon

1 tbsp olive oil

1 tsp sherry vinegar

We've based this recipe on a traditional Iranian classic known as kuku sabzi. There are many different versions but all contain loads of herbs, giving the omelette a wonderful green colour. We've included some potatoes and leave them unpeeled for extra fibre. Lovely with the tomato salad for a quick lunch.

Bring a pan of water to the boil, add the potatoes and blanch them for 1 minute, then drain and set aside.

Heat the olive oil in a deep frying pan and add the potatoes and onion. Fry until the onion is translucent and the potato is just cooked through but firm.

Put the herbs in a food processor with a splash of water and pulse until very finely chopped. Add the garlic and herbs to the frying pan and cook, stirring regularly, until the herbs have collapsed down a little. Preheat a grill to a medium heat.

Beat the eggs with the spices and season with salt and pepper. Stir them into the frying pan along with the barberries and almonds. Make sure everything is evenly distributed, then leave the omelette to cook until the bottom is set, then place the pan under the grill. Cook for just 2–3 minutes until the top is just set.

Leave the omelette to cool for a few minutes before attempting to turn it out – you might need to go round the edge with a palette knife first.

For the tomato salad, season the tomatoes with salt and pepper and toss them in the lemon zest and juice, olive oil and sherry vinegar. Serve with the omelette.

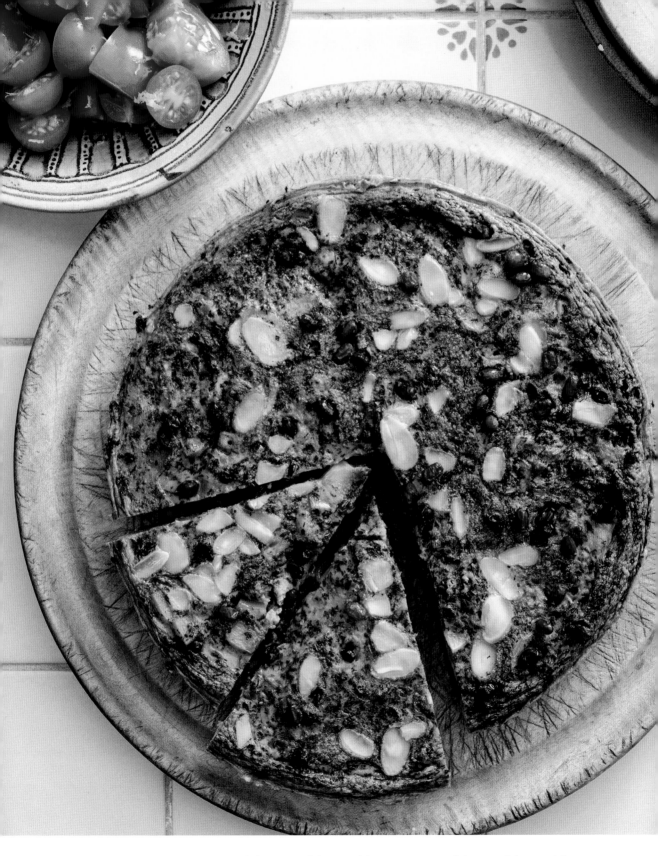

INFO PER SERVING: PROTEIN (G) 14.5   CARBS (G) 14   SUGAR (G) 7.5   FAT (G) 19   SATURATED FAT (G) 4   FIBRE (G) 3   SALT (G) 0.4

Serves: **4**

 Prep: **5 minutes**

 Cooking time:
about 15 minutes

 Calories per serving:
553

PASTA WITH CHILLI & LENTILS

400g spaghetti or linguini

3 tbsp olive oil

6 garlic cloves, very finely sliced

½ tsp chilli flakes, plus extra to serve

250g cooked brown or green lentils

small bunch of parsley, finely chopped

25g vegetarian Parmesan-style cheese, grated

salt

Spaghetti aglio e olio (spaghetti with garlic oil) is an Italian classic and one of our favourite pasta dishes. For this version, we decided to dress things up a little, adding some lentils for protein and chilli flakes for a hit of heat.

Bring a large pan of water to the boil and add salt, then the spaghetti or linguini. When the pasta is al dente, ladle off some of the cooking water and set it aside, then drain the pasta.

While the pasta is cooking, heat the oil in a large sauté pan and add the garlic. Cook the garlic very gently, making sure it doesn't take on any colour, then add the chilli flakes and a ladleful of the pasta cooking water to form a sauce.

Add the cooked pasta and lentils to the sauté pan. Toss to coat everything in the sauce and add a little more of the cooking water if it's looking dry. Sprinkle in most of the parsley and cheese and toss to coat again.

Serve with the remaining parsley and cheese and offer extra chilli flakes at the table for those who want more heat.

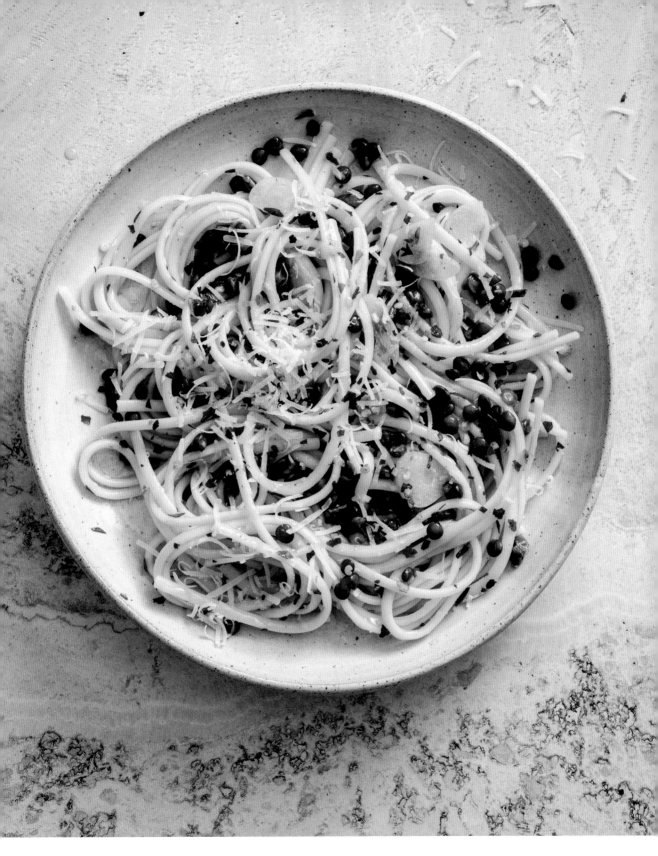

INFO PER SERVING: PROTEIN (G) 21.5   CARBS (G) 84   SUGAR (G) 2.5   FAT (G) 13   SATURATED FAT (G) 3   FIBRE (G) 9   SALT (G) 0.2

Serves: **4**

Prep: **10–15 minutes**

Cooking time:
about 30 minutes

Calories per serving:
410

SQUASH & QUINOA RISOTTO

1 tbsp olive oil

2 leeks, finely chopped

200g butternut squash, finely
   diced

3 garlic cloves, finely chopped

150g kale or cavolo nero, finely
   chopped

200g quinoa, soaked for
   5 minutes and drained

100ml white wine

600ml vegetable stock

1 tsp dried thyme or 1 tbsp
   fresh thyme leaves

400g can of cannellini beans,
   drained

35g vegetarian Parmesan-
   style cheese, grated, plus
   extra to serve

lemon juice

salt and black pepper

Quinoa is a real superfood. It's actually a seed not a grain, so is gluten-free, and it's high in protein and nutrients. We're using it here to make a hearty risotto-style dish that's packed with great veg and also contains some beans for extra bulk and protein. A very satisfying supper.

Heat the oil in a large sauté pan. Add the leeks and squash and stir them over a low heat until the leeks start to look glossy and translucent. Add the garlic and kale or cavolo nero and stir until the leaves have collapsed down, then stir in the quinoa. Season with salt and pepper.

Pour in the white wine and bring to the boil. When most of the wine has boiled off, add all the stock and sprinkle in the thyme, then bring back to the boil. Cover the pan, turn down the heat and simmer for 15–20 minutes, stirring regularly, until most of the liquid has been absorbed by the quinoa.

Roughly mash half the beans, then stir these and the whole beans into the quinoa. Leave to stand, covered, over a low heat for a further 5 minutes, then beat in the grated cheese.

Serve with a little more cheese and a squeeze of lemon juice.

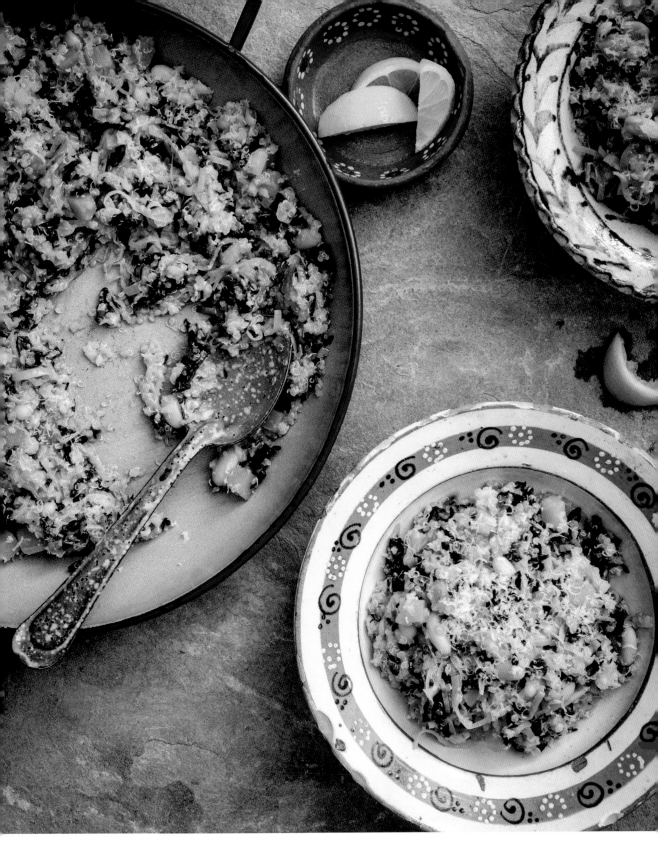

INFO PER SERVING: PROTEIN (G) 18   CARBS (G) 44   SUGAR (G) 9   FAT (G) 14   SATURATED FAT (G) 3   FIBRE (G) 12   SALT (G) 0.4

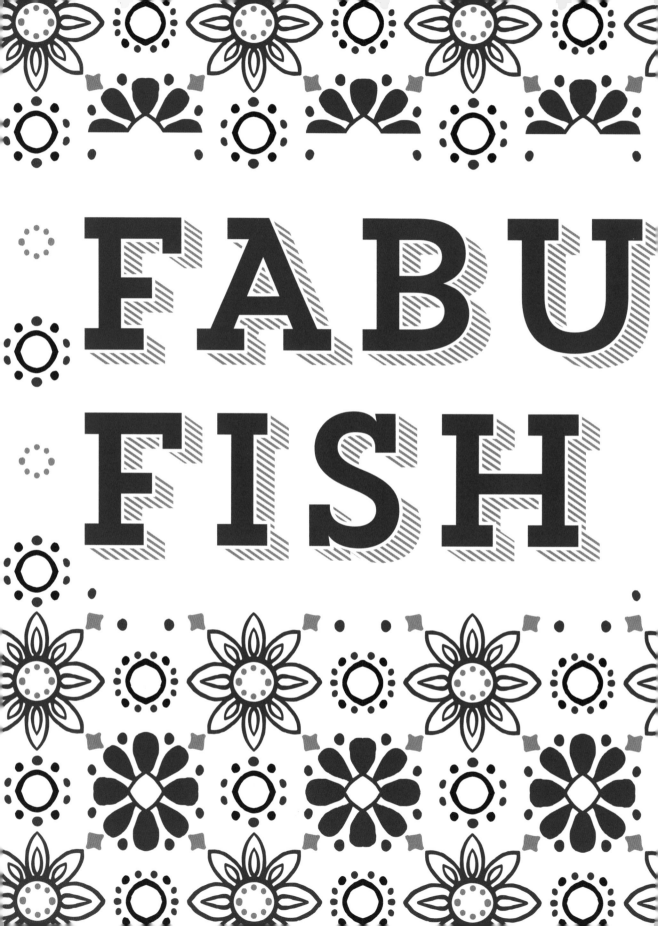

LOUS

ORECCHIETTE WITH CAVOLO NERO & HARISSA

TUNISIAN SPICY PASTRIES

SALMON & WATERCRESS FISHCAKES

FISH BRAISED WITH POTATOES, PEAS & BEANS

MACKEREL NIÇOISE

FINNISH FISH CHOWDER

GRILLED SARDINES WITH SALSA

MUSSELS WITH RED WINE, CHILLI & POTATOES

SMOKED FISH & SWEETCORN

SPICY SHRIMP CREOLE

MEDITERRANEAN FISH TRAY BAKE

Serves: **4**

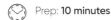 Prep: **10 minutes**

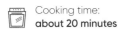 Cooking time:
about 20 minutes

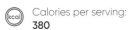 Calories per serving:
380

ORECCHIETTE WITH CAVOLO NERO & HARISSA

1 tbsp olive oil

1 red onion, finely chopped

1 small tin of anchovies

3 garlic cloves, finely chopped

150g cavolo nero or similar,
    destemmed and shredded

100g canned chopped
    tomatoes

1 tbsp harissa paste

300g orecchiette pasta

800ml vegetable or chicken
    stock or water

salt and black pepper

TO SERVE

grated Parmesan (optional)

This is one of those crafty pasta dishes that's cooked all in one pot – and we do love a one-pot. You could make it veggie by leaving out the anchovies, but they do add protein and a lovely savoury flavour. And, of course, anchovies are an oily fish and we should all be eating more of those. The harissa brings a nice whack of heat to complete the dish. Orecchiette means 'little ears' and you can see why!

Heat the olive oil in a large saucepan. Add the onion and sauté over a medium-high heat until it's starting to take on some colour. Add the anchovies, along with their oil, breaking them up with a wooden spoon, then stir in the garlic and cavolo nero. Stir until the cavolo nero has wilted down a little, then add the tomatoes and 2 teaspoons of the harissa paste.

Stir in the orecchiette and pour the stock or water into the pan, making sure the orecchiette is pushed under the liquid as much as possible. Season with salt and pepper and bring to the boil, then turn down the heat to somewhere between a boil and a simmer and cover the pan. Cook for about 15 minutes, stirring every so often, until the orecchiette and the cavolo nero are tender.

Taste for seasoning and heat, then stir in the remaining harissa paste if you want to ramp up the heat. Serve with grated Parmesan if you like.

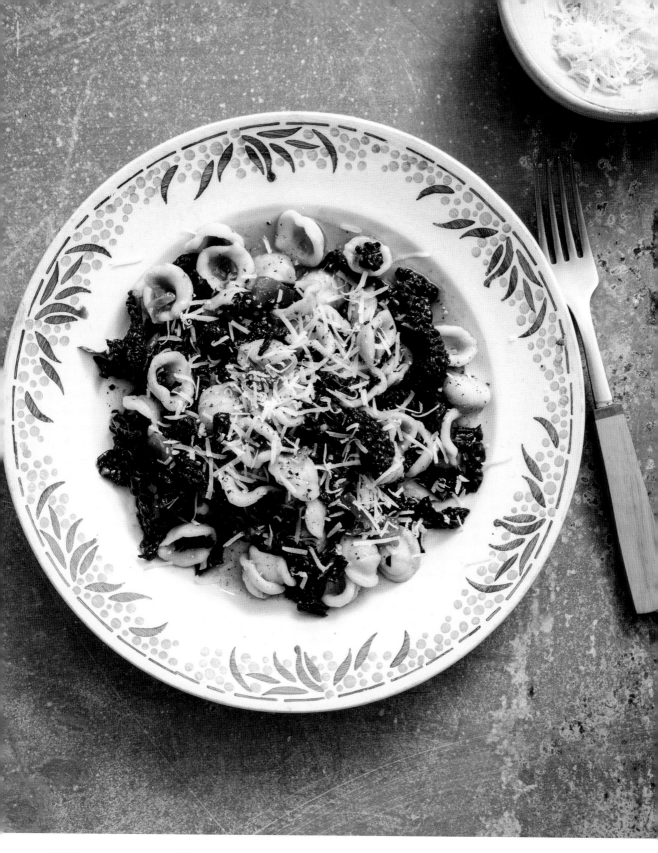

INFO PER SERVING: PROTEIN (G) 15   CARBS (G) 60   SUGAR (G) 6.5   FAT (G) 7   SATURATED FAT (G) 1.5   FIBRE (G) 7   SALT (G) 2.5

Serves: **4**

 Prep: **20 minutes**

 Cooking time:
8–11 minutes

 Calories per pastry:
428

TUNISIAN SPICY PASTRIES

olive oil

1 pack of filo pastry

1 egg, beaten, for brushing

4 eggs

FILLING

350g cooked potato, crushed

3 spring onions, finely chopped

2 tbsp capers, rinsed

160g can of tuna, drained
(112g drained weight)

small bunch of parsley, finely
chopped

small bunch of coriander,
finely chopped

½ tsp ground turmeric

salt and black pepper

TO SERVE

chilli sauce (optional)

In North African countries these savoury treats are made with a very light thin pastry known as brick or brik. You can buy it in the UK, but you can also use filo instead which is readily available in supermarkets. Use leftover mash in the filling or the flesh from a couple of baked potatoes – we tend to leave the skin on and just crush it roughly for extra fibre and texture. Seriously good and if you want a veggie version, just leave out the tuna.

Preheat the oven to 200°C/Fan 180°C/Gas 6. Brush 2 baking sheets with olive oil.

Put all the filling ingredients in a bowl and mix them together thoroughly. Season with plenty of salt and pepper.

Cut the sheets of filo into squares, each measuring about 25 x 25cm. Filo often comes in packs of 7 sheets, and you need 8 for this recipe so you might have to make the last square up from a couple of offcuts.

Take a square of filo and brush it with beaten egg. Lay another square on top. Take a quarter of the filling and arrange it over one triangular half of the filo. Make a well in the middle of the filling and drop an egg into the well – the filling will hold the egg in place. Season the egg with salt and pepper. Brush the edges of the remaining half of the pastry with more beaten egg, then fold it over and seal. Place the parcel carefully on to one of the baking sheets and brush with olive oil. Repeat with the remaining squares of filo, filling and eggs.

Bake the parcels in the preheated oven until the pastry is crisp and golden and the eggs are just cooked. How long you leave them depends on how you want the eggs cooked. For a runny yolk and just set whites, cook for 8 minutes for a medium egg or 9 minutes for a large egg. Increase the cooking time to 10–11 minutes for a set yolk.

Serve piping hot, with some chilli sauce if you like.

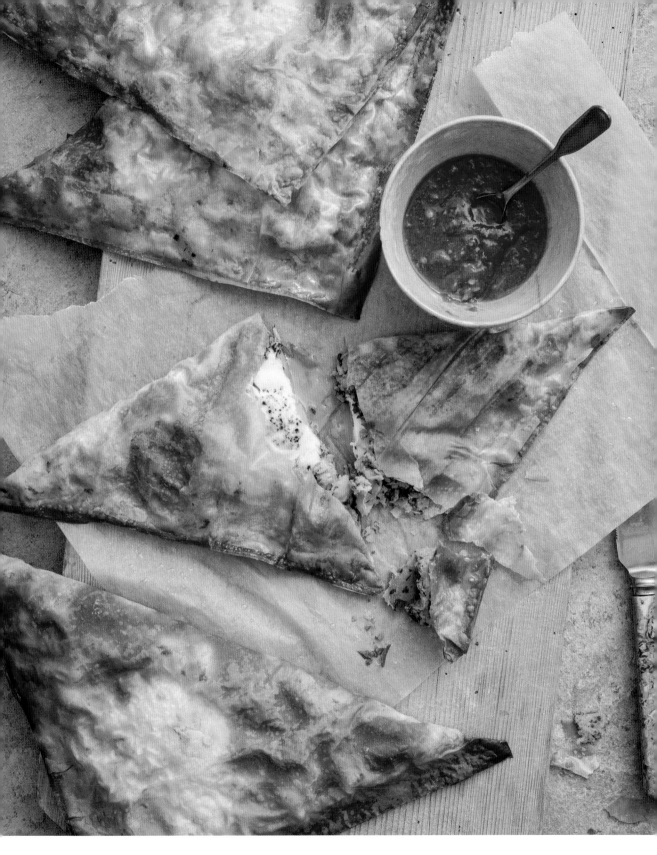

INFO PER PASTRY: PROTEIN (G) 25   CARBS (G) 54   SUGAR (G) 3   FAT (G) 12   SATURATED FAT (G) 2.5   FIBRE (G) 5   SALT (G) 1.4

Serves: **4**

 Prep: **15 minutes, plus chilling time**

 Cooking time: **about 30 minutes**

 Calories per serving: **517**

SALMON & WATERCRESS FISHCAKES

600g skinned salmon fillet

1 tbsp olive oil

1 shallot, very finely chopped

75g watercress sprigs (no thick, woody stems), chopped

zest of 1 lime

2 tsp Dijon mustard

250g mashed potato

1 tbsp plain flour, for dusting

2 tbsp olive oil for frying

salt and black pepper

SAUCE

150g yoghurt or kefir

1 tsp Dijon mustard

juice and zest of ½ lime

fronds from a small bunch dill, finely chopped

Salmon and peppery watercress make the perfect combo for these fishcakes – great protein and lots of lovely flavour from the watercress. We decided to drop all the business of dipping them in egg and breadcrumbs, both to reduce the work and the calorie count. Just dusting them with flour is fine. And you could also make these with tinned salmon or the hot smoked stuff you sometimes see in the shops. If you don't want to fry the fishcakes, you can bake them in the oven. Brush them with oil, then cook in a preheated oven at 200°C/Fan 180°C/Gas 6, for 15 minutes.

Season the fish with salt and pepper, then put it in a saucepan – try to make it a snug fit so you don't have to use too much water. Cover the fish with cold water, put a lid on the pan and bring to the boil. Remove the pan from the heat and leave to stand for 5 minutes. The fish will be just cooked through.

Remove the fish from the cooking liquor and leave it to cool. Flake the flesh into a bowl, checking for any stray bones as you go.

Heat the olive oil in a small frying pan, then add the shallot and sauté until it's translucent. Add the watercress and stir until it has wilted, then remove from the pan and leave to cool.

Add the watercress and shallot mixture to the fish, then add the lime zest, mustard and mashed potato. Season with salt and pepper and mix thoroughly. Shape into 8 fishcakes and chill thoroughly.

Dust the fishcakes with flour. Heat a tablespoon of olive oil in a large frying pan and add the fishcakes – you may have to cook them in a couple of batches. Fry them for 3–4 minutes on each side until a crust has developed.

To make the sauce, mix everything together and season with salt and pepper. Serve the fishcakes with the sauce.

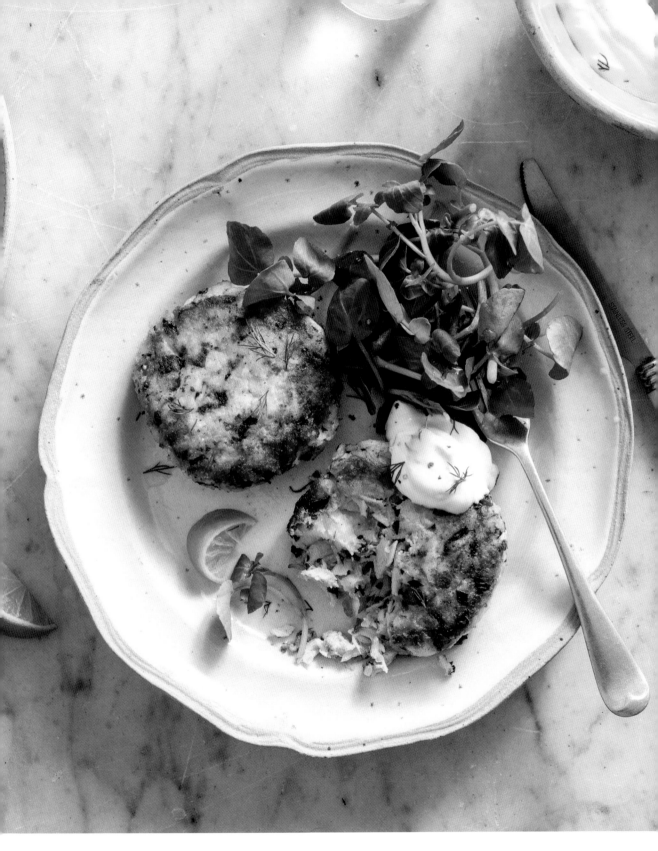

Serves: **4**

 Prep: **10–15 minutes**

 Cooking time:
about 30 minutes

 Calories per serving:
400

1 tbsp olive oil

15g butter

2 leeks, thickly sliced

500g baby potatoes, sliced
   if large

1 courgette, sliced into rounds

3 garlic cloves, finely chopped

leaves from 2 large tarragon
   sprigs, finely chopped

150ml white wine

200g frozen peas, defrosted

200g frozen broad beans,
   defrosted

4 x 150g white fish fillets

zest of 1 lemon

salt and black pepper

FISH BRAISED WITH POTATOES, PEAS & BEANS

Here's another fab one-pot – fish, carbs and loads of lovely veg. And if you're nervous about cooking fish, it's very simple to make too. Cooking time for the fish depends on the thickness – a very thin fillet of basa or bass will only take about three minutes, while a thicker piece of cod or hake will need five or six minutes.

Heat the olive oil and butter in a large, lidded sauté pan or a shallow flameproof casserole dish. When the butter has melted, add the leeks, potatoes and courgette and season with salt and pepper. Stir to coat the vegetables with the oil and butter, then add the garlic and tarragon and pour the wine into the pan. Bring to the boil, then turn down the heat and cover the pan. Leave everything to braise gently for about 15 minutes until the potatoes are completely cooked through.

Add the peas and broad beans. Cover the pan again and leave to cook gently for another 5 minutes. Season the fish fillets with salt and pepper and sprinkle over the lemon zest. Place the fish fillets on top of the vegetables and cover. Place over a low heat for a few minutes or until the fish is just cooked through.

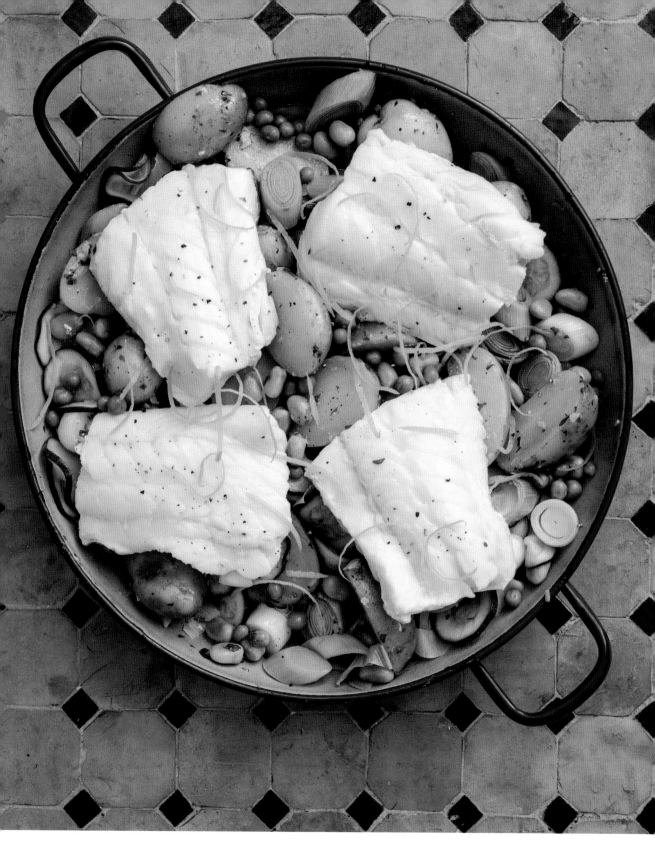

INFO PER SERVING: PROTEIN (G) 37   CARBS (G) 31   SUGAR (G) 6   FAT (G) 9   SATURATED FAT (G) 3   FIBRE (G) 12   SALT (G) 0.4

Serves: **4**

 Prep: **15 minutes**

 Cooking time:
about 15 minutes

 Calories per serving:
473

MACKEREL NIÇOISE

200g salad potatoes, sliced
    if large

100g green beans, trimmed

4 little gem lettuces, trimmed
    and quartered lengthways

4 medium tomatoes, quartered

2 roasted red peppers, pulled
    into strips

2 smoked mackerel fillets,
    skinned and pulled into
    chunks

4 eggs, hard-boiled and
    quartered

50g pitted black olives

25g capers, drained

a few basil leaves

a few thyme leaves (optional)

DRESSING

2 tbsp olive oil

1 tbsp red wine vinegar

1 tbsp Dijon mustard

1 garlic clove, crushed

With this, we're taking a Niçoise salad to another level with the addition of some smoked mackerel which is available in every supermarket. Oily fish, lots of veg and protein – what's not to love? You could also use other smoked fish or tinned sardines. We think this makes a cracking lunch on a summer's day, or any day really.

Bring a saucepan of water to the boil and add plenty of salt, then drop in the potatoes. Boil for 6–7 minutes until they're just about tender to the point of a knife, then add the green beans. Cook for a further 2–3 minutes, until the beans are al dente. Drain and run the beans under cold water to cool and retain their fresh green colour. Set both the beans and potatoes aside while you make the dressing.

Whisk the dressing ingredients together and add a little water to thin it if necessary, then season with salt and pepper.

To assemble, arrange the little gems over a large serving platter. Add the potatoes, green beans and tomatoes. Season with salt and pepper.

Drape over the strips of red pepper, followed by the mackerel chunks. Drizzle over half the dressing and toss very gently. Top with the eggs, olives and capers.

Add the remaining dressing and finish with the basil and the thyme leaves, if using.

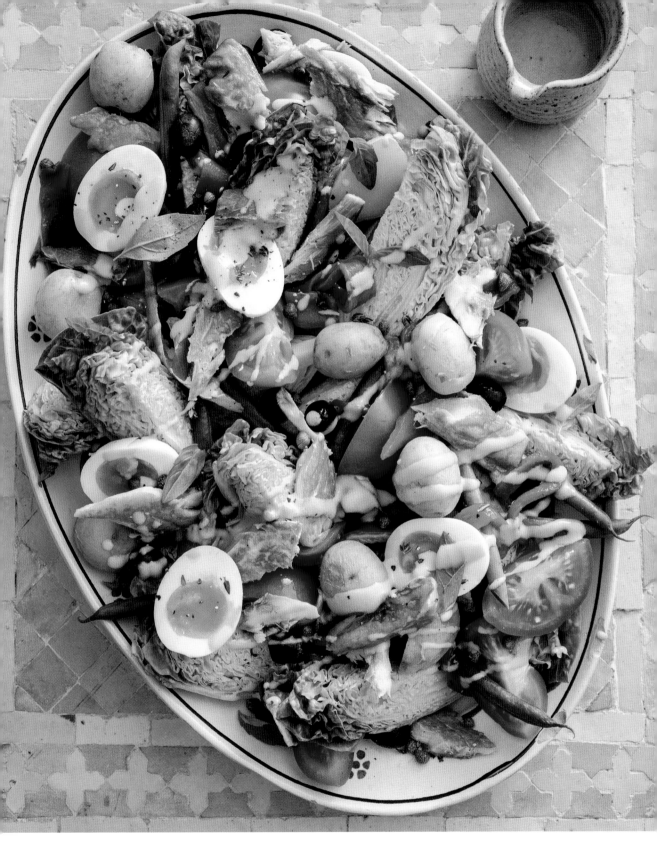

INFO PER SERVING: PROTEIN (G) 27   CARBS (G) 16.5   SUGAR (G) 8   FAT (G) 32   SATURATED FAT (G) 6.5   FIBRE (G) 5.5   SALT (G) 2.3

Serves: **4**

 Prep: **10–15 minutes**

 Cooking time:
about 25 minutes

 Calories per serving:
350

FINNISH FISH CHOWDER

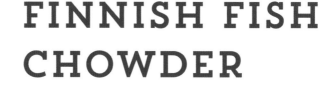

1 tbsp olive oil

5g butter

2 leeks, finely sliced

1 celery stick, sliced

1 large carrot, thinly sliced
    on the diagonal

300g potatoes (unpeeled),
    diced

2 garlic cloves, finely chopped

2 bay leaves

1 tsp ground allspice

a small bunch of dill

800ml fish or vegetable stock
    or water

600g white fish fillets, cut into
    chunks

100ml whipping cream

salt and black pepper

Everyone loves a chowder and we've based this recipe on a soup I enjoyed while on a trip to Finland. We've made it slightly healthier than usual by cutting down on the butter and using a bit of olive oil. The potatoes are good but you could also use celeriac for a slightly different flavour. Nice with any kind of white fish. (Dave)

Heat the olive oil and butter in a large saucepan. Add the leeks, celery, carrot and potatoes, and stir until they're all coated in the oil and butter. Add the garlic, bay leaves and allspice, then stir again for a minute.

Separate the dill fronds from the thicker stems. Bundle the stems up together and add them to the pan. Pour in the stock and season with salt and pepper.

Bring to the boil, then turn down the heat to a simmer and partially cover the pan. Leave to cook for about 15 minutes until the vegetables are tender.

Add the fish and the cream to the saucepan and simmer for another 2–3 minutes until the fish is just cooked through. Roughly chop the dill fronds and add them to the soup. Remove the bay leaves and serve immediately.

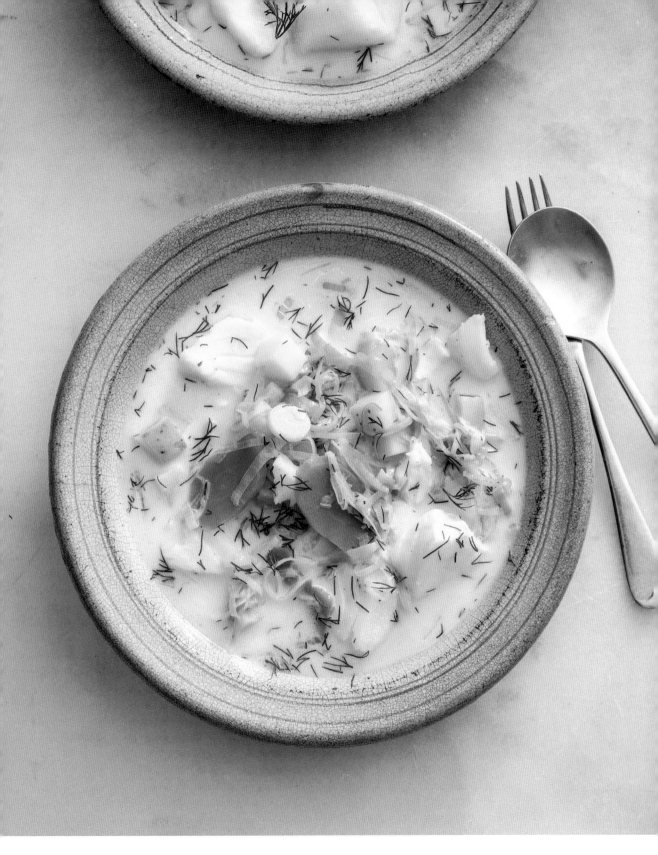

INFO PER SERVING: PROTEIN (G) 30 CARBS (G) 19 SUGAR (G) 5 FAT (G) 16 SATURATED FAT (G) 8 FIBRE (G) 5 SALT (G) 0.5

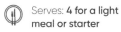 Serves: **4 for a light meal or starter**

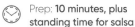 Prep: **10 minutes, plus standing time for salsa**

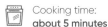 Cooking time: **about 5 minutes**

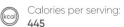 Calories per serving: **445**

GRILLED SARDINES WITH SALSA

12–16 sardines (depending on size), butterflied
1 tbsp olive oil
salt and black pepper

SALSA
1 small red onion, very finely chopped
1 tbsp sherry vinegar
zest of 1 lemon
2 medium tomatoes, finely diced
small bunch of parsley, finely chopped
½ tsp hot paprika

Sardines are cheap and super nutritious – we should all be eating more oily fish – and this makes a great quick meal if you can buy ready-butterflied sardines at the fish counter. It's not that hard to butterfly them yourself, but why give yourself the extra work? Serve the sardines with our little salsa for a light meal that's low in carbs and high in protein and good fats.

First, put the red onion for the salsa in a bowl, sprinkle it with salt and add the sherry vinegar. Leave it to stand for half an hour, then add all the remaining ingredients and season with pepper.

Heat your grill to its highest setting. Rub the sardines with olive oil and sprinkle them with salt and pepper. Arrange the sardines on a rack, skin-side up, then grill them for 4–5 minutes, turning the rack around once, until the skins are lightly browned in places and the fish are cooked through.

Serve the sardines with the salsa.

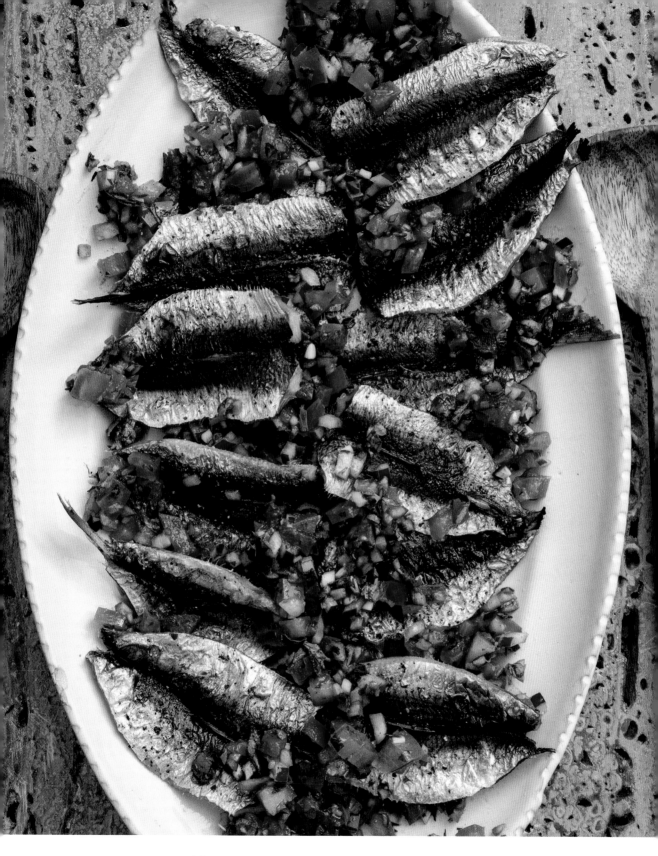

INFO PER SERVING: PROTEIN (G) 60   CARBS (G) 3   SUGAR (G) 3   FAT (G) 21   SATURATED FAT (G) 6   FIBRE (G) 1   SALT (G) 1

Serves: **4**

 Prep: **20 minutes**

 Cooking time:
about 25 minutes

 Calories per serving:
223

MUSSELS WITH RED WINE, CHILLI & POTATOES

1kg mussels (or one net)

1 tbsp olive oil

1 red onion, sliced into wedges

1 red pepper, cut into strips

300g baby new potatoes, sliced

3 garlic cloves, finely chopped

2 red chillies, finely sliced into rounds

200ml red wine

300ml chicken or vegetable stock

200g chopped tomatoes (fresh or canned)

1 large thyme sprig

2 bay leaves

1 tsp dried oregano

salt and black pepper

TO SERVE

leaves from a small bunch of parsley

½ tsp chilli flakes (optional)

Let's eat more mussels! They are cheap to buy, packed with protein and a real treat to eat. In this recipe, we've combined them with potatoes and other veg to make a complete meal in a bowl. With a hit of chilli and the richness of red wine, this is lip-smackingly good.

Wash the mussels thoroughly and pull off any beards. Discard any that don't close when sharply tapped.

Heat the olive oil in a large saucepan or a flameproof casserole dish with a lid. Add the red onion, red pepper and potatoes. Sauté until everything has taken on a bit of colour, then add the garlic and chillies. Stir for another couple of minutes.

Add the red wine and bring to the boil. Allow the wine to bubble furiously until reduced by half, then add the stock, tomatoes, thyme, bay leaves and oregano. Season with salt and pepper. Bring to the boil again, then turn the heat down and cover the pan. Simmer for about 15 minutes until the potatoes are tender and the flavours have had a chance to blend.

Turn up the heat again and add the mussels to the pan. Cover and cook the mussels for 3–4 minutes, shaking the pan regularly. The mussels are ready when they have fully opened – remove and discard any that remain closed.

Taste for seasoning and serve the mussels in shallow bowls. Add a sprinkling of parsley and some chilli flakes, if using.

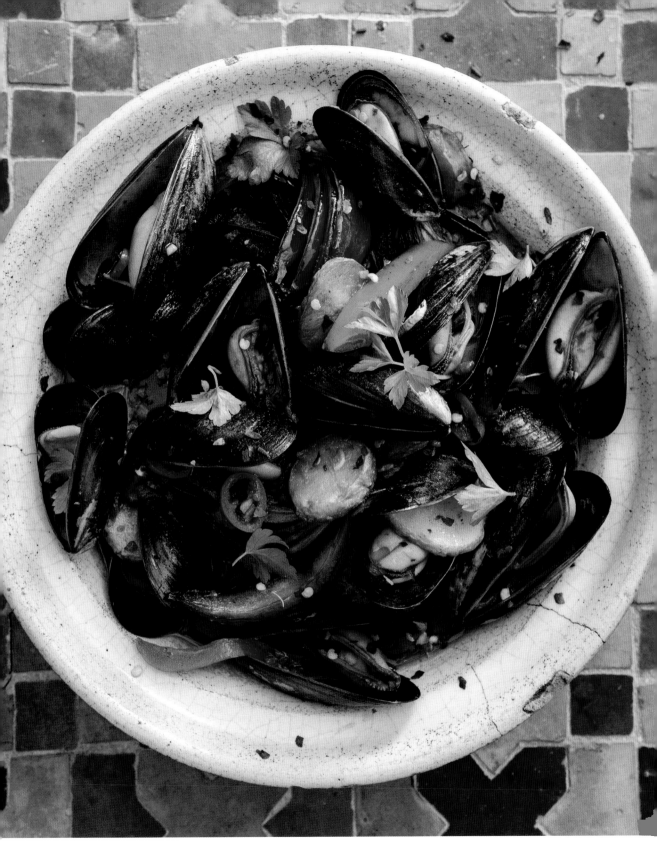

INFO PER SERVING: PROTEIN (G) 17 CARBS (G) 18 SUGAR (G) 6 FAT (G) 4.5 SATURATED FAT (G) 1 FIBRE (G) 3.5 SALT (G) 0.6

Serves: **4**

 Prep: **10 minutes**

Cooking time:
about 30 minutes

Calories per serving:
432

SMOKED FISH & SWEETCORN

1 tbsp olive oil

400g potatoes, sliced

2 leeks, sliced

1 red pepper, sliced

3 garlic cloves, finely chopped

200ml fish or chicken stock

1 tsp chipotle paste or similar

1 tsp dried oregano

400g sweetcorn

2 tbsp crème fraiche

200g cherry tomatoes

4 x 150g smoked white fish
fillets

50g Cheddar, grated

salt and black pepper

This dish is proper comfort food and everything you need in one pan. Just watch the cooking time for the fish – thin fillets will only take about 3 minutes or so but give thicker pieces a bit longer. Easy to make, this is a warming and tasty meal.

Heat the olive oil in a large, ovenproof dish – a ceramic or enamelled cast-iron one is best. Add the potatoes, leeks, red pepper and garlic. Stir to coat them all with the oil and season with salt and pepper. Whisk the stock with the chipotle paste and pour this over the vegetables. Sprinkle over the oregano and stir.

Bring to the boil and cover the dish with a lid or foil. Turn down the heat and simmer until the vegetables are tender, then stir in the sweetcorn and crème fraiche. Dot the cherry tomatoes over the top.

Preheat your grill. Season the fish fillets with salt and pepper and place them on top of the vegetables, then sprinkle with the cheese. Cover the dish again and cook over a low heat for several minutes to cook the fish and tomatoes – the thicker the fillets the longer they will take to cook. Uncover the dish and place under the hot grill to brown the cheese.

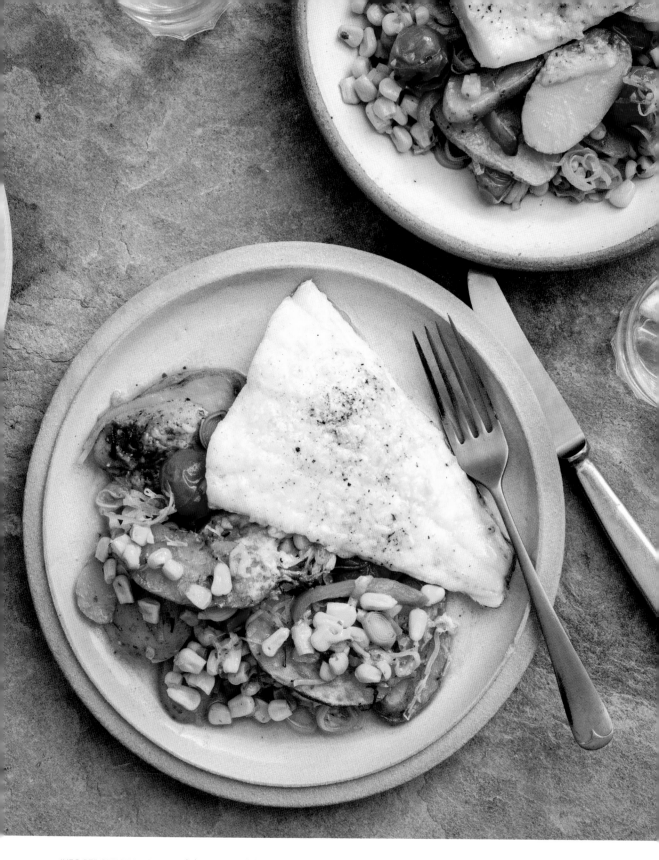

INFO PER SERVING: PROTEIN (G) 41   CARBS (G) 32   SUGAR (G) 8   FAT (G) 14   SATURATED FAT (G) 6   FIBRE (G) 8   SALT (G) 1.9

Serves: **4**

 Prep: **15 minutes**

 Cooking time:
35–40 minutes

 Calories per serving
(without rice): **213**

SPICY SHRIMP CREOLE

400g large, peeled shrimp,
   deveined
zest and juice of 1 lemon
2 tbsp olive oil
1 large onion, diced
2 celery sticks, diced
1 green pepper, diced
1 red pepper, diced
3 garlic cloves, finely chopped
400g can of chopped
   tomatoes
200ml vegetable stock
1 tsp Worcestershire sauce
5g butter
handful of parsley, finely
   chopped
salt and black pepper

SPICE MIX
1 tsp hot paprika
1 tsp garlic powder
1 tsp onion powder
1 tsp ground white pepper
1 tsp dried oregano
1 tsp dried thyme

We first ate this cracking dish in the great city of New Orleans where it's a local favourite. And, just like the best Mediterranean recipes, it's rich in seafood and veg, with the addition of plenty of spices. If you prefer, of course, you could use a Creole seasoning mix instead of making your own.

Toss the shrimp in the lemon zest and some ground black pepper and set aside. Mix all the ingredients for the spice mix together and set aside.

Heat the olive oil in a large flameproof casserole dish or a sauté pan and ddd the onion, celery and peppers. Cook over a high heat for a couple of minutes, then turn down the heat and cover the pan. Leave to cook for at least 5 minutes or as long as 10, stirring regularly, until the onion and celery are translucent and everything is tender to the point of a knife, .

Add the garlic and the spice mix to the pan and stir for a couple of minutes, then add the tomatoes. Rinse out the can with the stock, then add this to the pan too. Add the Worcestershire sauce and season with salt and pepper. Bring to the boil, then turn down the heat and cover the pan. Cook for 10 minutes, then remove the lid and cook for a further 5 minutes to reduce the sauce.

Heat the butter in a separate frying pan, add the shrimp and cook until pink. Stir the shrimp into the sauce, then add lemon juice to taste. Sprinkle with chopped parsley, then serve with some rice if you like.

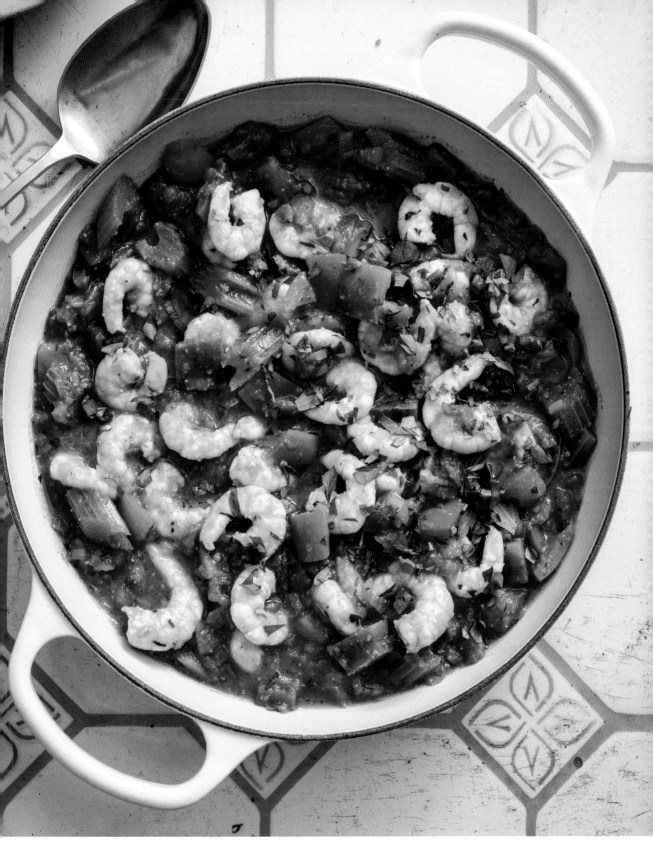

INFO PER SERVING: PROTEIN (G) 22 CARBS (G) 11 SUGAR (G) 10 FAT (G) 8 SATURATED FAT (G) 2 FIBRE (G) 4 SALT (G) 1.6

Serves: **4**

 Prep: **10–15 minutes**

 Cooking time:
about 35 minutes

 Calories per serving:
470

MEDITERRANEAN FISH TRAY BAKE

3 red onions, cut into wedges

3 red peppers, cut into thick
   strips

1 fennel bulb, cut into wedges

2 tbsp olive oil

1 tsp dried oregano or mixed
   herbs

100ml white wine

400g can of cannellini beans,
   drained

1 courgette, cut into slices

200g sprouting broccoli

4 x 100g salmon fillets

2 tbsp capers, drained

a few basil leaves

zest of ½ lemon

salt and black pepper

We know that salmon isn't a Mediterranean fish, but it works well in a tray bake, is readily available and, like all oily fish, is rich in nutrients. So, we've dressed it up with a bit of Mediterranean style and veg and got a great result. Another all-in-one supper.

Preheat the oven to 200°C/Fan 180°C/Gas 6.

Put the onions, peppers and fennel into a large roasting tin and drizzle with half the olive oil. Sprinkle over half the dried herbs and season with salt and pepper. Roast in the preheated oven for 15 minutes.

Pour in the white wine and add the cannellini beans. Give the tin a good shake so the beans spread around the vegetables. Put the courgette and broccoli in a bowl and sprinkle over the rest of the olive oil. Toss until well coated, then arrange over the vegetables in the roasting tin and roast for a further 10 minutes.

Season the salmon fillets with salt and pepper. Place them on top of the vegetables, skin-side down, and sprinkle over the remaining herbs, followed by the capers. Roast for another 7–8 minutes until the salmon is just cooked.

Remove from the oven and garnish with a few basil leaves. Grate some lemon zest over the salmon before serving.

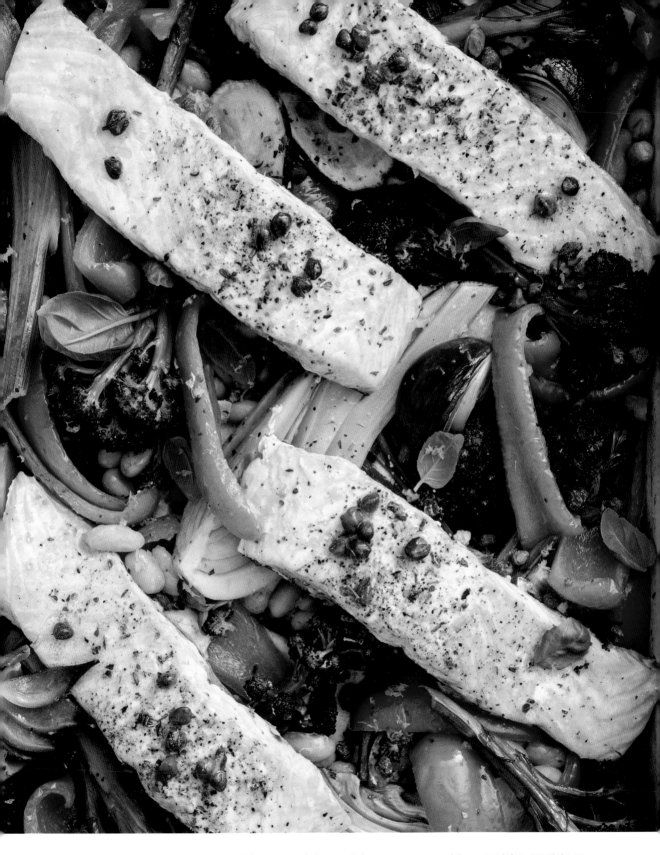

CHIC & ME

MEDITERRANEAN CHICKEN STIR-FRY
PULLED CHICKEN TACOS
GREEK-STYLE GRILLED CHICKEN
CHICKEN & VEGETABLE CURRY
AUTUMN CHICKEN TRAY BAKE
PASTA WITH MEATBALLS & CHARD
PORK STEAKS WITH GRAPES &
 MUSTARD

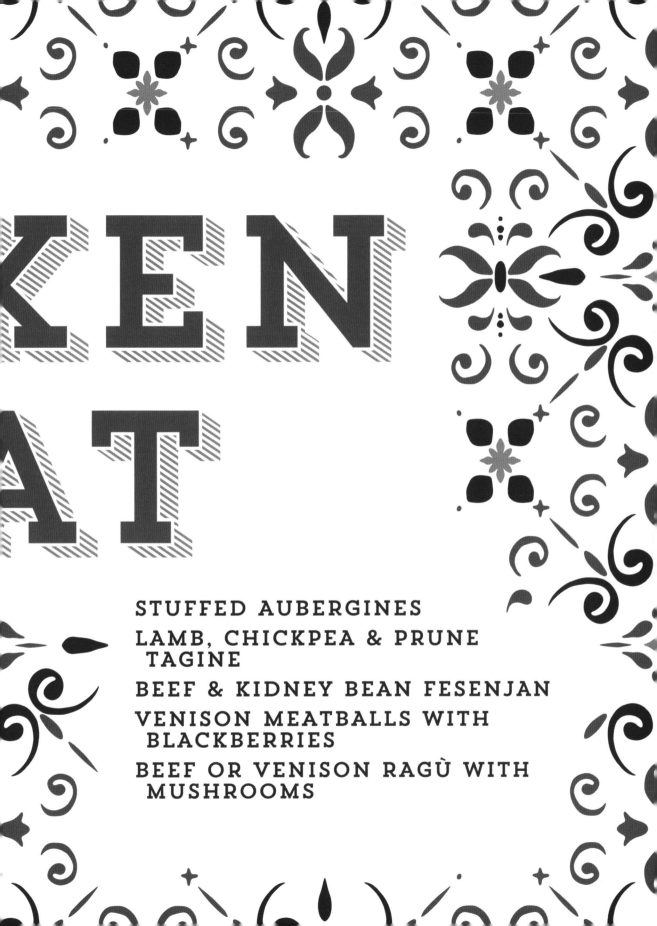

STUFFED AUBERGINES

LAMB, CHICKPEA & PRUNE TAGINE

BEEF & KIDNEY BEAN FESENJAN

VENISON MEATBALLS WITH BLACKBERRIES

BEEF OR VENISON RAGÙ WITH MUSHROOMS

Serves: **4**

 Prep: **15 minutes**

 Cooking time:
about 20 minutes

 Calories per serving:
328

MEDITERRANEAN CHICKEN STIR-FRY

500g boneless chicken breast
or thigh meat, skinned and
finely sliced
zest and juice of ½ lemon
1 tsp dried mint
1 tsp dried oregano
2 tbsp olive oil

VEGETABLES

200g green beans, trimmed
250g sprouting broccoli,
trimmed
1 red onion, sliced into wedges
1 red pepper, cut into strips
2 courgettes, cut on the
diagonal
3 garlic cloves, finely chopped
250g cherry tomatoes, halved
1–2 tsp sherry or red wine
vinegar
salt and black pepper

TO SERVE

50g black olives, pitted
1 orange, segmented
a few mint and basil leaves

Some fabulous fusion going on here. We're taking Mediterranean ingredients and cooking them stir-fry style for a quick, super-tasty meal. One tip: don't be tempted to skip the blanching step for the beans and broccoli, as they need that bit of extra cooking. To make this veggie, you could use griddled halloumi instead of chicken.

Toss the chicken in the lemon zest, juice and dried herbs. Heat a tablespoon of the oil in a large sauté pan or wok. When it's hot, add the chicken and stir-fry until lightly browned and just cooked through. Remove it with a slotted spoon and set aside.

Bring a saucepan of water to the boil and add the green beans and broccoli. Blanch for 2 minutes, then strain and refresh under cold water.

Heat the remaining olive oil in your pan or wok. Add the red onion, red pepper and courgettes and stir-fry until they are the crisp side of al dente. Add the blanched green beans and broccoli and the garlic, then continue to cook until the vegetables are almost tender to the point of a knife.

Fold the chicken through the vegetables, add the cherry tomatoes and continue to stir-fry until the tomatoes have warmed through. Season with salt and pepper. Drizzle in half the vinegar and taste, then adjust the seasoning and add more vinegar if necessary. Serve sprinkled with the olives, orange segments and herbs. This is nice on its own or you could serve with rice or couscous.

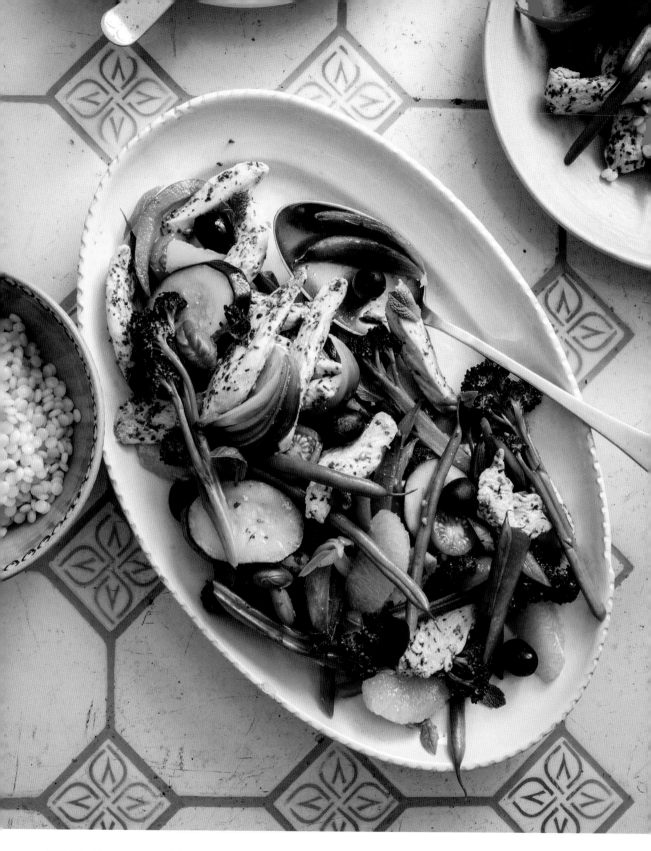

INFO PER SERVING: PROTEIN (G) 36.5   CARBS (G) 15.5   SUGAR (G) 11   FAT (G) 11.5   SATURATED FAT (G) 2   FIBRE (G) 8   SALT (G) 0.6

Makes: **12**

 Prep: **15 minutes**

 Cooking time:
about 15 minutes

 Calories per taco: **237**

PULLED CHICKEN TACOS

1 tbsp olive oil

2 medium red onions, cut into
   slim wedges

2 red peppers, sliced into strips

3 garlic cloves, finely chopped

2 tsp chipotle paste

1 tbsp tomato purée

2 cooked chicken breasts,
   pulled into long strips

salt and black pepper

SPICE MIX (or use 1 tbsp
   of taco seasoning)

½ tsp dried oregano

½ tsp ground cumin

½ tsp ground coriander

½ tsp garlic powder

½ tsp ground cinnamon

½ tsp ground allspice

TO SERVE

2 avocados

zest and juice of 1 lime

a small bunch of coriander,
   finely chopped

12 corn tortillas

2 tbsp finely chopped pickled
   jalapeños (optional)

Here's a speedy feast that all the family will enjoy. We suggest topping the tacos just with diced avocado and jalapeños to keep the calories down, but if you feel like going wild, you could throw caution to the wind and serve them with a good dollop of soured cream and some grated cheese.

If making the spice mix, combine all the ingredients and stir well, then set aside.

Heat the oil in a large sauté pan and add the onions and peppers. Sauté over a high heat until they are starting to brown and just al dente. Stir in the garlic and sprinkle over the spice mix.

Whisk the chipotle paste and tomato purée with 150ml of water and pour it over the vegetables. Add the chicken to the pan and season with salt and pepper. Bring to the boil and simmer, uncovered, until the liquid has reduced.

Peel and dice the avocados, then toss them with half a teaspoon of salt, the lime zest and juice and the coriander. Warm the tortillas and load them with the chicken. Top with avocado and the jalapeños, if you want extra heat.

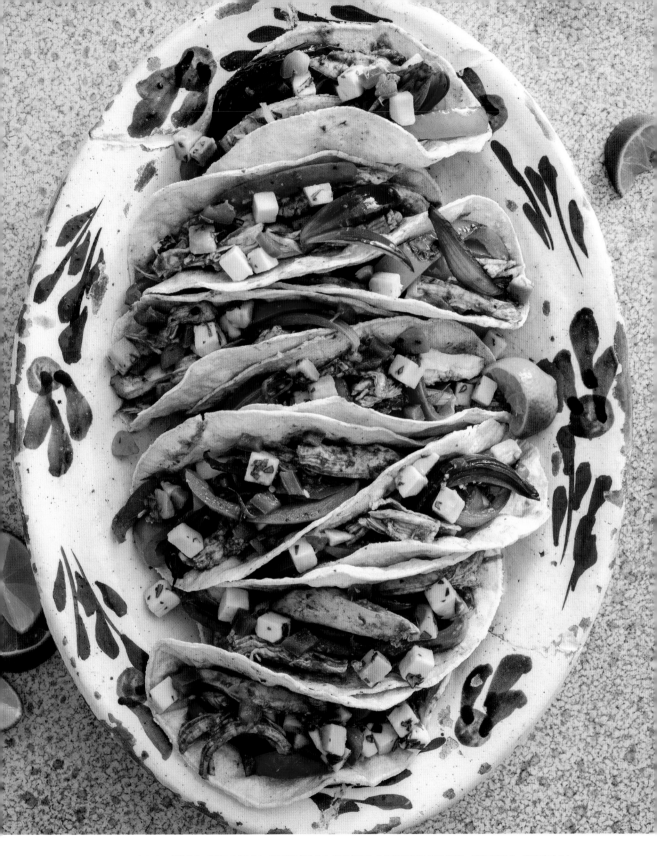

INFO PER TACO: PROTEIN (G) 11.5 CARBS (G) 26 SUGAR (G) 3.5 FAT (G) 9 SATURATED FAT (G) 2 FIBRE (G) 3 SALT (G) 0.4

Serves: **4**

 Prep: **10 minutes, plus marinating time**

 Cooking time: **about 15 minutes**

 Calories per serving (with tzatziki): **324**

GREEK-STYLE GRILLED CHICKEN

4 chicken breasts, skinned and butterflied

3 tbsp olive oil

zest of 1 lemon

1 large rosemary sprig, finely chopped

leaves from a thyme sprig, bruised

leaves from a large oregano sprig, chopped or
1 tsp dried oregano

salt and black pepper

TZATZIKI

½ large cucumber

250g Greek yoghurt or thick kefir

1 small garlic clove, very finely chopped

2 tsp dried mint

Butterflying the chicken breasts, so they are half the thickness, helps them cook quickly and stay moist and tender. This dish brings back memories of lunches in the sun but it's great at any time of year. Serve with some tzatziki and a salad, such as the beetroot salad on page 176.

Season the chicken with salt and black pepper. Put the olive oil in a bowl with the lemon zest and herbs. Add the chicken breasts to the bowl and rub the herby oil into the flesh. Leave to marinate for at least an hour or cover the bowl and leave in the fridge for several hours or overnight.

For the tzatziki, cut the cucumber in half lengthways and scoop out the seeds. Coarsely grate the cucumber and sprinkle it with salt, then leave to stand in a colander for half an hour. Gently squeeze out any excess liquid.

Put the cucumber in a bowl with the yoghurt or kefir, the garlic and the dried mint. Stir to combine and season with salt and pepper.

When you are ready to cook the chicken, heat a griddle pan. Scrape off any excess marinade from the chicken. When the griddle is too hot to hold your hand over, place the chicken on it and grill for 2–3 minutes on each side until char lines appear and the chicken is cooked through. Best to do this in a couple of batches so you don't overcrowd the pan. Serve the chicken with the tzatziki.

TIP

To butterfly a chicken breast, place it on your work surface. Take a sharp knife and insert it along the long side of the breast. Slice into the breast, but stop just short of the other side. Open out the breast like a book.

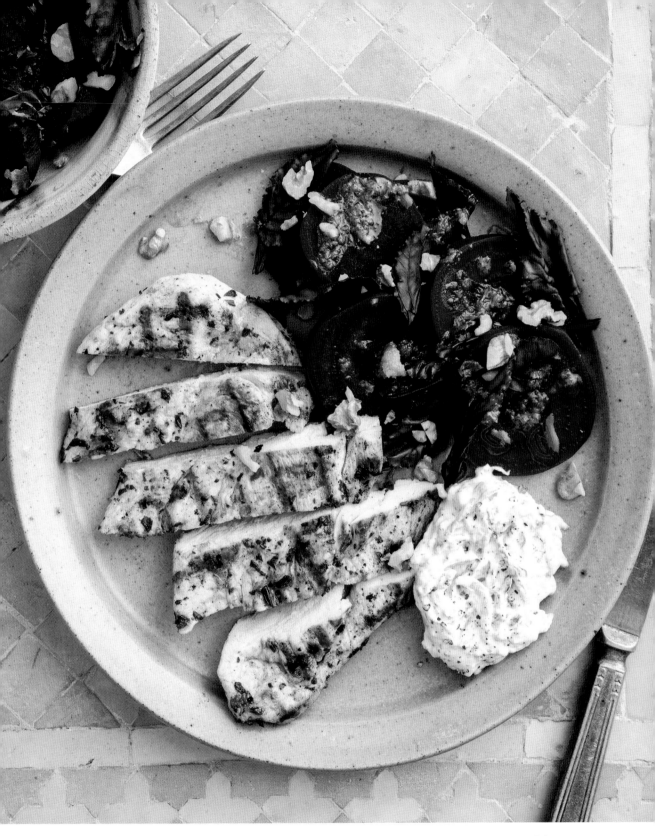

INFO PER SERVING (WITH TZATZIKI):   PROTEIN (G) 40   CARBS (G) 3.5   SUGAR (G) 3   FAT (G) 17   SATURATED FAT (G) 8
FIBRE (G) 0.5   SALT (G) 0.3

Serves: **4**

 Prep: **15 minutes**

 Cooking time:
about 25 minutes

 Calories: **242**

CHICKEN & VEGETABLE CURRY

1 large bunch of coriander, stems and leaves separated

1 tsp coconut oil

1 onion, thickly sliced

4 boneless chicken thighs, skinned and diced

1 aubergine, cut into 3cm chunks

3 garlic cloves, finely chopped

1 tbsp medium curry powder

200g coconut milk

200g green beans, trimmed

juice of ½ lime

200g medium tomatoes, cut into quarters

3 green chillies, finely sliced (optional)

salt and black pepper

A fresh, fragrant curry, this recipe is more about the herbs and the vegetables than spices and makes a few chicken thighs go a long way. It's good on its own or with some flatbread or rice. Why not try this on a Friday night instead of ordering a takeaway?

Finely chop the coriander stems and most of the leaves, keeping them separate. Set aside some of the leaves to garnish the curry.

Heat the coconut oil in a large saucepan or a flameproof casserole dish and add the onion, chicken and aubergine. Stir over a high heat until everything has taken on a little colour, then add the garlic, coriander stems and curry powder. Stir for a minute or so, then pour in the coconut milk. Season with salt and pepper.

Bring to the boil, then turn down the heat and simmer for 10 minutes until the chicken is cooked through and the aubergines are tender. Add the green beans and continue to cook until just al dente.

Blitz most of the coriander leaves with a little water and the lime juice, then add this to the pan along with the tomatoes. Simmer for a few more minutes, uncovered, until the tomatoes have softened.

Serve garnished with the reserved coriander leaves and the green chillies, if using.

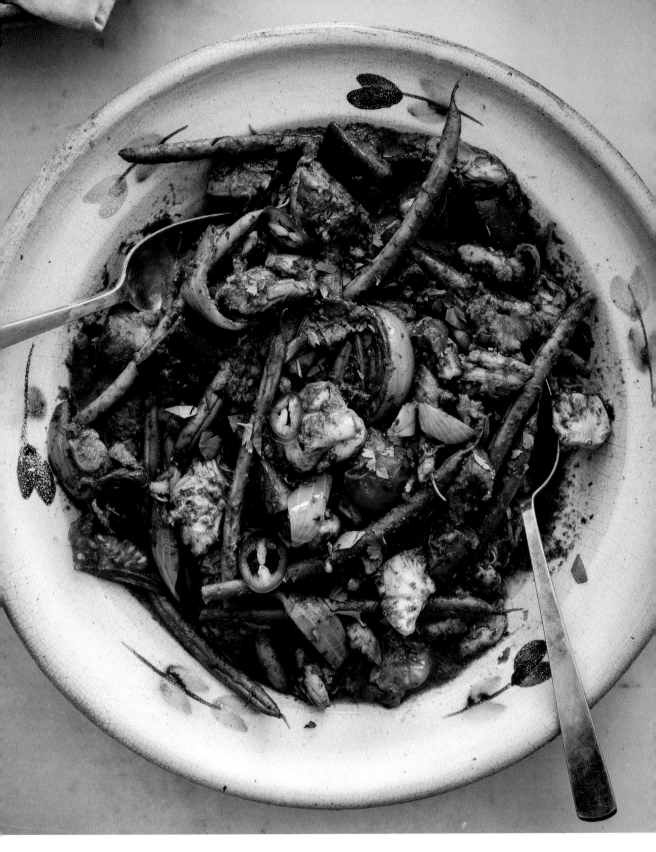

INFO PER SERVING: PROTEIN (G) 19 CARBS (G) 10 SUGAR (G) 7 FAT (G) 12 SATURATED FAT (G) 9 FIBRE (G) 7 SALT (G) 0.2

Serves: **4**

 Prep: **15 minutes**

 Cooking time:
40–45 minutes

 Calories per serving:
349

AUTUMN CHICKEN TRAY BAKE

3 carrots, cut into thick batons

3 leeks, cut into chunks

1 small red cabbage, cut into
    wedges

2 tbsp olive oil

100ml white wine

100ml chicken stock

1 tbsp wholegrain mustard

2 bay leaves

250g chestnut mushrooms,
    left whole

100g cooked chestnuts
    (vacuum packed), left whole

6 skinless chicken thigh fillets,
    cut in half

1 tsp rubbed sage

salt and black pepper

A tray bake always makes a great family meal. It takes very little time to put together, then you can leave the oven to work its magic while you get on with having fun. Chestnuts and mushrooms give this recipe an autumnal vibe and the wine, stock and mustard combine to make a nice bit of sauce.

Preheat the oven to 200°C/Fan 180°C/Gas 6.

Put the carrots, leeks and red cabbage into a large roasting tin and drizzle over a tablespoon of the olive oil. Season with salt and pepper and mix thoroughly. Whisk the white wine with the chicken stock and mustard. Pour this around the vegetables and add the bay leaves. Cover the tin with foil and bake in the oven for 20 minutes.

Remove the foil. Add the chestnut mushrooms and chestnuts to the roasting tin. Put the chicken in a bowl and drizzle over the remaining oil. Season with salt and pepper and sprinkle with the sage, then mix well so the chicken is nicely coated. Add the chicken to the roasting tin.

Roast for a further 20–25 minutes, uncovered, until everything is cooked and the sauce has thickened. Serve with a big pile of steamed greens.

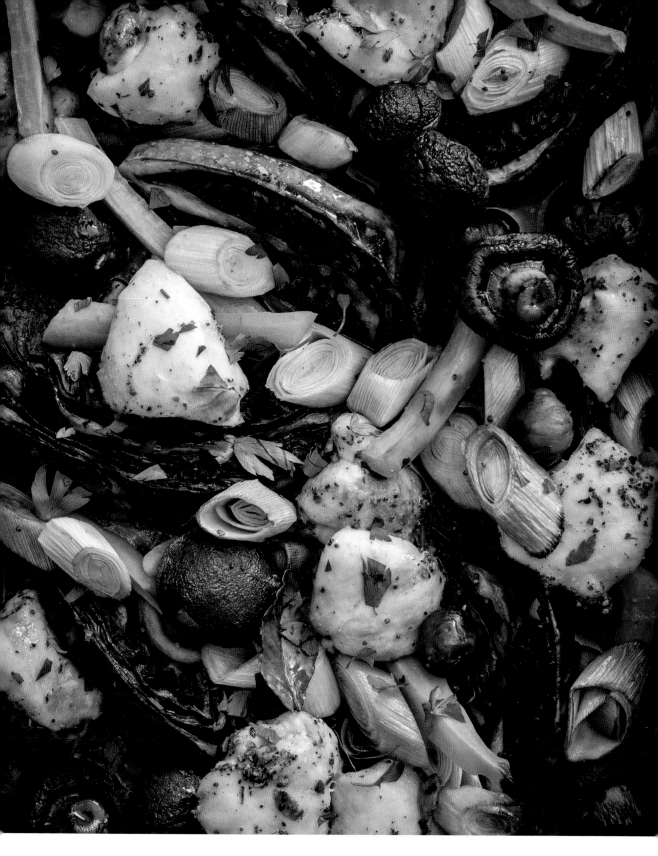

INFO PER SERVING: PROTEIN (G) 31 CARBS (G) 21 SUGAR (G) 13.5 FAT (G) 11 SATURATED FAT (G) 2 FIBRE (G) 12 SALT (G) 0.6

Serves: **4**

 Prep: **15 minutes**

 Cooking time:
35–40 minutes

 Calories per serving:
722

PASTA WITH MEATBALLS & CHARD

A good hearty dish, this one is a bit higher in calories and carbs than most of the recipes in this book, but it makes a great family supper. Our meatballs are dead tasty but if you really want a quick meal you could use shop-bought meatballs. Just don't tell anyone.

MEATBALLS

400g minced pork

1 garlic clove, crushed
    or grated

zest of 1 lemon

½ tsp fennel seeds

½ tsp chilli powder

40g wholemeal breadcrumbs

1 egg

2 tbsp olive oil

salt and black pepper

PASTA & SAUCE

1 onion, finely chopped

200g chard, stems and leaves
    separated, finely chopped

2 garlic cloves, finely chopped

100ml white wine

400g short pasta, such
    as penne

100g cream cheese

lemon juice

First make the meatballs. Mix all the ingredients, except the oil, together and season with salt and pepper, then form the mixture into 16 balls. Heat a tablespoon of the oil in a large frying pan. When the oil is hot, add the meatballs. Sear them on the underside, being careful not to turn them until they lift off the pan cleanly, then sear them on the other side. Remove them from the pan and set aside.

Heat the remaining oil in a large saucepan and add the onion and chard stems. Sauté them until softened and translucent, then add the garlic. Cook for another couple of minutes, then stir in the chard leaves. When they have wilted down, add the white wine. Let it boil for a couple of minutes, then add the meatballs and season with salt and pepper. Cover the pan and leave to simmer for 10 minutes until the meatballs are completely cooked through.

In another pan, cook the pasta in plenty of salted water, then drain, reserving a couple of ladlefuls of the cooking water.

Mix the cream cheese with enough of the reserved pasta cooking water to give it the texture of double cream, then add this and the pasta to the pan of meatballs and chard. Simmer for a couple of minutes to make sure everything is piping hot, adding a little more of the cooking water if necessary. Add a squeeze of lemon juice and season with plenty of pepper, then serve.

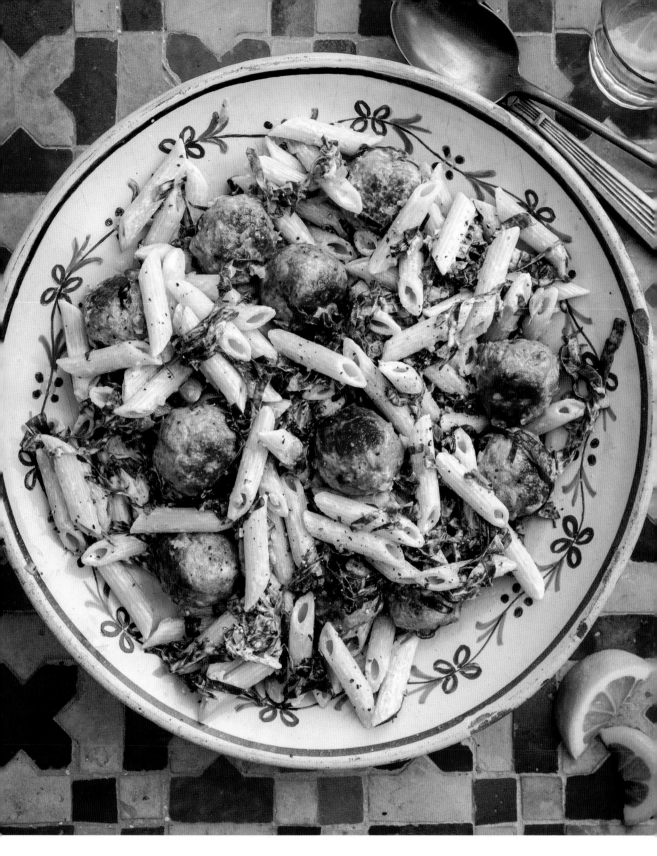

INFO PER SERVING: PROTEIN (G) 37   CARBS (G) 81.5   SUGAR (G) 6   FAT (G) 24   SATURATED FAT (G) 9   FIBRE (G) 6.5   SALT (G) 0.8

Serves: **4**

 Prep: **10 minutes**

 Cooking time:
about 30 minutes

 Calories per serving:
269

PORK STEAKS WITH GRAPES & MUSTARD

1 tbsp olive oil

4 thin pork steaks or escalopes

1 onion, thinly sliced

1 garlic clove, finely chopped

30 red grapes

a few sage leaves, finely
chopped

150ml white wine

2 tsp Dijon mustard

2 tsp red wine or sherry vinegar

150ml chicken stock or water

a few parsley leaves, finely
chopped

salt and black pepper

The inspiration for this recipe is the much-loved Italian condiment known as mostarda, which is basically fruit in a mustard-flavoured syrup. We've taken those flavours to make a sauce for pork and it's a big success. Serve with some green veg.

Heat the olive oil in a large sauté pan. Season the pork steaks with salt and pepper, then fry them for a couple of minutes on each side until well browned. Remove from the pan and set aside.

Add the onion and sauté over a medium-high heat until it is starting to soften, then add the garlic and grapes. Continue to sauté until the grape skins start to take on some colour and wrinkle. Stir in the sage leaves.

Pour in the white wine and bring to the boil. Deglaze the pan with the wine, then stir in the mustard, vinegar and stock or water. Season and bring to the boil. Simmer until the liquid is reduced by about a third, then put the pork steaks back in the pan along with any juices and warm them through for a minute. Serve the pork with the sauce and garnish with the parsley.

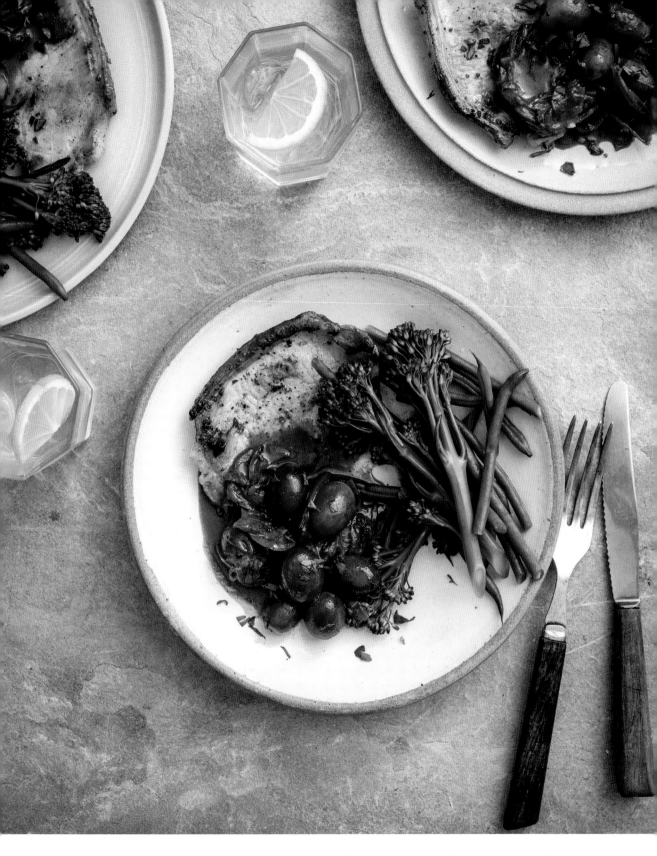

INFO PER SERVING: PROTEIN (G) 35 CARBS (G) 6 SUGAR (G) 5.5 FAT (G) 8 SATURATED FAT (G) 2.5 FIBRE (G) 1 SALT (G) 0.5

Serves: **4**

 Prep: **15 minutes**

 Cooking time:
**about 1 hour and
10 minutes**

 Calories per serving:
455

STUFFED AUBERGINES

4 medium aubergines

2 tbsp olive oil

300g lamb mince

1 onion, finely chopped

1 red pepper, diced

2 garlic cloves, finely chopped

1 tbsp ras-el-hanout

1 tsp dried mint

400g can of chickpeas,
   drained

200g chopped tomatoes
   (canned are fine)

zest and juice of ½ lemon

salt and black pepper

TOPPING (OPTIONAL)

100g halloumi, coarsely grated

leaves from a small bunch
   parsley, finely chopped

1 preserved lemon, very finely
   chopped

Stuffed aubergines are popular all over the Med and Middle Eastern regions, and like many Mediterranean dishes they do a good job of making the most of a small amount of meat. We're really pleased with this latest version and we do recommend using the halloumi and preserved lemon topping – it's sensational.

Preheat the oven to 200°C/Fan 180°C/Gas 6. Cut the aubergines in half lengthways, then use a sharp knife to score cross-hatching through the flesh of each half. Brush the aubergines with olive oil and season with salt.

Place the aubergines in a couple of roasting tins and roast them in the oven for 35–40 minutes until lightly browned and fairly soft but not completely tender.

Meanwhile, cook the filling. Heat a frying pan and add the lamb mince. Let it sear on the underside before breaking it up and browning it all over – it will start rendering out fat very quickly. When the base of the pan is coated with some of the fat, add the onion and red pepper and sauté over a medium heat for 5 minutes. Stir in the garlic, ras-el-hanout and mint, then season with salt and pepper.

Add the chickpeas and tomatoes along with 200ml of water, then bring to the boil. Turn down the heat and simmer, uncovered, until everything is tender and the sauce has reduced.

Scoop out the flesh from the aubergines, leaving a relatively thick layer behind – about ½ cm. Roughly chop the scooped-out flesh and add it to the lamb, together with the lemon zest and juice. Cook for a further 5 minutes, then taste a little of the mixture to check the seasoning and adjust as necessary.

Spoon the filling into the aubergines. If using the topping, mix the halloumi with two-thirds of the parsley and all of the preserved lemon and sprinkle over the top of the aubergines. Put the aubergines back in the oven for another 10 minutes until piping hot, then serve sprinkled with the remaining chopped parsley.

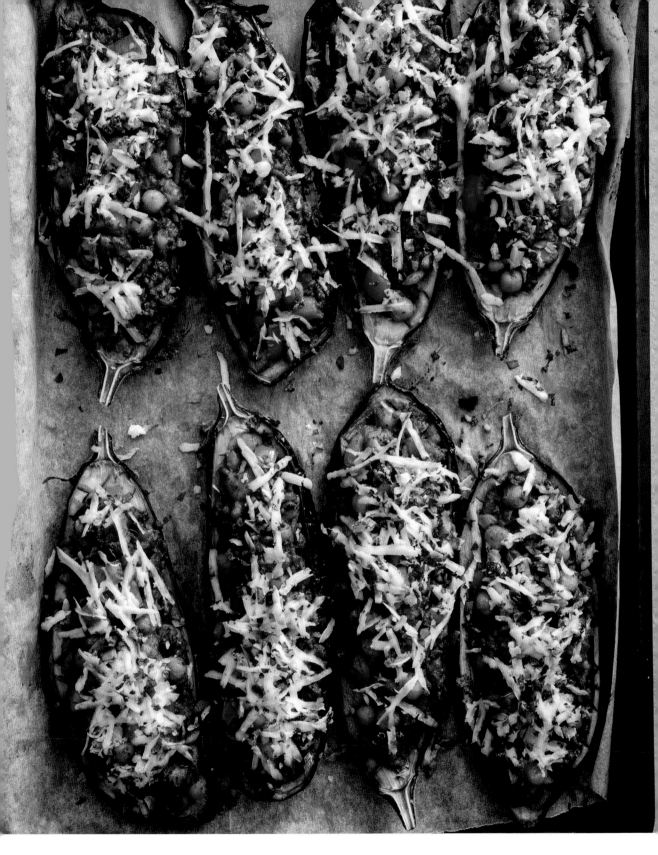

INFO PER SERVING: PROTEIN (G) 29 CARBS (G) 23 SUGAR (G) 12 FAT (G) 25 SATURATED FAT (G) 10 FIBRE (G) 14 SALT (G) 1.6

Serves: **4**

 Prep: **15 minutes**

 Cooking time:
1 hour and 15 minutes

 Calories per serving:
540

LAMB, CHICKPEA & PRUNE TAGINE

1 tbsp olive oil

600g lamb neck fillet, trimmed of fat and cut into chunks

2 small red onions, cut into wedges

2 carrots, sliced on the diagonal

3 garlic cloves, finely chopped

1 tbsp ras-el-hanout

400g can of chopped tomatoes

400ml chicken, lamb or vegetable stock

pinch of saffron, soaked in a little warm water

400g can of chickpeas, drained

100g pitted prunes

200g green beans

a squeeze of lemon juice

leaves from a few parsley sprigs, finely chopped (optional)

salt and black pepper

A tantalisingly tasty tagine, this dish does have to be cooked for a while, but you can prepare it ahead up to the point when the lamb is cooked. Then it can be set aside until you're ready to add the saffron, chickpeas and so on. The advantage to doing this is that if the lamb is left to cool, the fat will set on the top and can be skimmed off before finishing the dish. This is good recipe to make if entertaining friends, as most of the work can be done in advance. Ras-el-hanout, by the way, is a North African spice mix that's traditionally used in tagines. You can find it in supermarkets now.

Heat the olive oil in a large flameproof casserole dish or a saucepan. Season the lamb and sear it on both sides in the oil, then remove it from the pan and set aside.

Add the red onions and carrots and sear them until they have taken on some colour. Stir in the garlic and put the lamb back in the pan, then sprinkle in the ras-el-hanout and stir to coat the lamb. Pour in the tomatoes and stock and stir to make sure the base of the pan is deglazed. Season with salt and pepper, then bring to the boil, turn down the heat and partially cover the pan. Simmer for 45–50 minutes until the lamb is well on the way to being tender. You can prepare the dish ahead to this point.

Pour in the saffron and its water, then add the chickpeas, prunes and green beans. Cook until the beans are tender – up to another 10 minutes. Taste for seasoning and add a squeeze of lemon juice. Sprinkle with parsley, if using, then serve..

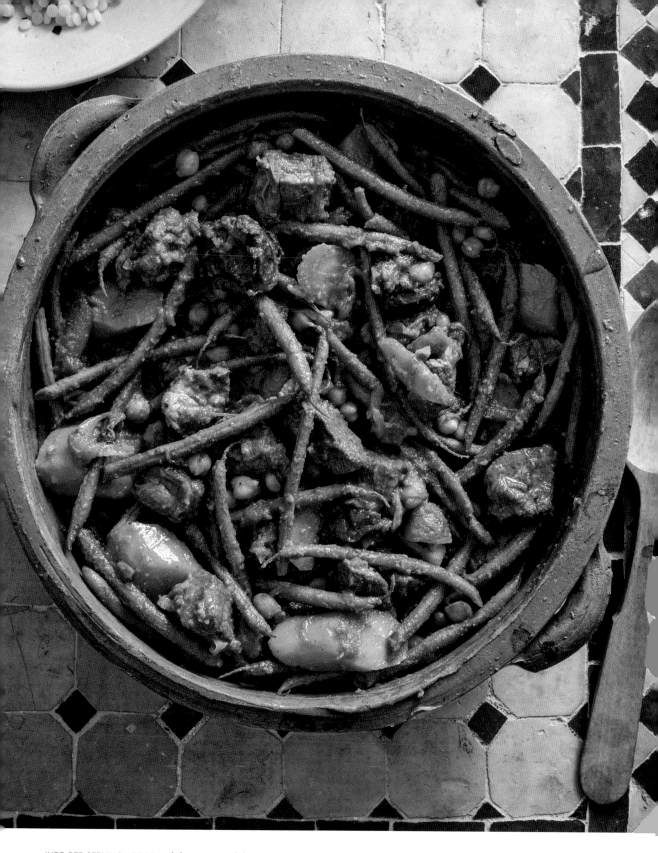

INFO PER SERVING: PROTEIN (G) 40   CARBS (G) 31   SUGAR (G) 20   FAT (G) 26   SATURATED FAT (G) 10.5   FIBRE (G) 11   SALT (G) 0.5

Serves: **4**

 Prep: **15 minutes**

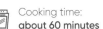 Cooking time:
about 60 minutes

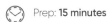 Calories per serving:
749

BEEF & KIDNEY BEAN FESENJAN

2 tbsp olive oil

500g braising or stewing steak, diced

1 large onion, thickly sliced

200g walnut halves

½ tsp cinnamon

large pinch of saffron, soaked in 2 tbsp warm water

400ml chicken stock

400g can of kidney beans, drained

100ml pomegranate molasses

1 tsp honey

salt and black pepper

TO GARNISH

a few parsley leaves

3 tbsp pomegranate seeds

A fesenjan is a traditional Persian dish of stewed meat with walnuts and pomegranate molasses, garnished with pomegranate seeds. It's luxurious and incredibly delicious. Just be careful grinding the walnuts so they don't end up as a paste – it's best to do a small amount at a time. This is good served with brown rice.

Heat a tablespoon of the oil in a large flameproof casserole dish with a lid. Season the beef with salt and pepper, then sear it quickly on all sides. Remove it from the pan and set aside, then add the remaining oil. Add the onion and cook until it is starting to soften.

Next grind the walnuts to the consistency of shop-bought ground almonds. To make sure you do this evenly without them starting to release oil and form a paste, grind a few at a time, using the pulse button on your food processor.

Add the walnuts to the onion with the cinnamon, then stir until the walnuts start to smell toasted. Put the beef back in the pan and stir to coat.

Add the saffron, stock and beans. Season with salt and black pepper, then bring to the boil and turn down the heat. Partially cover the pan and simmer for 30 minutes or so, until the beef is well on the way to becoming tender. Stir in the pomegranate molasses and honey, then continue to simmer, uncovered, until the sauce has thickened. Stir regularly during this time to make sure the mixture doesn't catch on the base of the pan.

Taste for seasoning and serve sprinkled with parsley and pomegranate seeds.

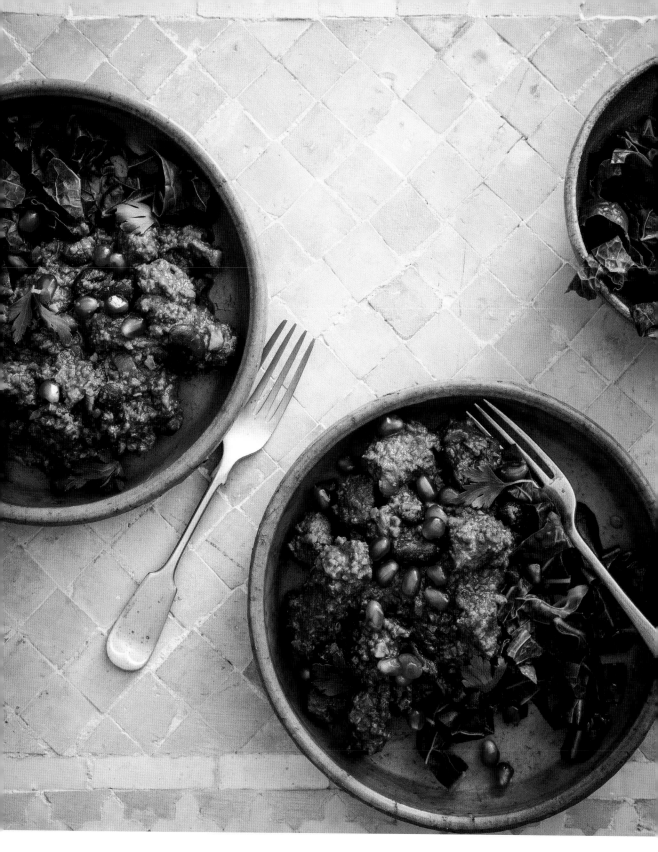

INFO PER SERVING: PROTEIN (G) 42.5   CARBS (G) 38   SUGAR (G) 20   FAT (G) 45.5   SATURATED FAT (G) 7   FIBRE (G) 9.5   SALT (G) 0.5

Serves: **4**

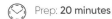 Prep: **20 minutes**

 Cooking time:
about 45 minutes

 Calories per serving
(without rösti): **327**

MEATBALLS

500g venison, minced

1 shallot, very finely chopped

50g wholemeal breadcrumbs

1 egg

1 tbsp crème fraiche

1 tsp Dijon mustard

½ tsp dried thyme

salt and black pepper

BRAISE

2 tbsp olive oil

1 large onion, finely chopped

15g dried mushrooms, soaked
  in warm water

3 garlic cloves, finely chopped

1 tsp juniper berries, lightly
  crushed

2 bay leaves

1 thyme sprig or 1 tsp dried
  thyme

150ml red wine

250ml chicken or mushroom
  stock

150g blackberries

1–2 tsp honey

VENISON MEATBALLS WITH BLACKBERRIES

Venison is a good, lean, healthy meat. It's available in many of the supermarkets now and we should probably be using it more often. Blackberries are a perfect partner for the meatballs and make a wonderful juicy sauce. Rösti (page 172) are a good accompaniment or you could serve the meatballs with celeriac or ordinary mash.

First make the meatballs. Put all the ingredients in a bowl and season with plenty of salt and pepper. Mix thoroughly, then form into 16–20 meatballs.

Heat a tablespoon of the oil in a large, lidded sauté pan or a shallow flameproof casserole dish. Add the meatballs and sear them on at least 2 sides, then remove them from the pan and set aside.

Add the remaining oil followed by the onion and sauté over a medium heat until the onion is a light golden brown. Strain the dried mushrooms and finely chop them, then add them to the onion along with the garlic, juniper berries and herbs. Stir for a minute, then pour in the red wine.

Bring the wine to the boil and cook furiously for a couple of minutes, stirring as you go to deglaze the base of the pan. Add the chicken or mushroom stock and season with salt and pepper.

Put the meatballs back in the pan. Bring to the boil again, then turn down the heat and simmer, partially covered, until the meatballs are cooked through and the sauce has reduced a little.

Stir in the blackberries and a teaspoon of the honey. Simmer for a couple of minutes, then taste and add more honey if you like.

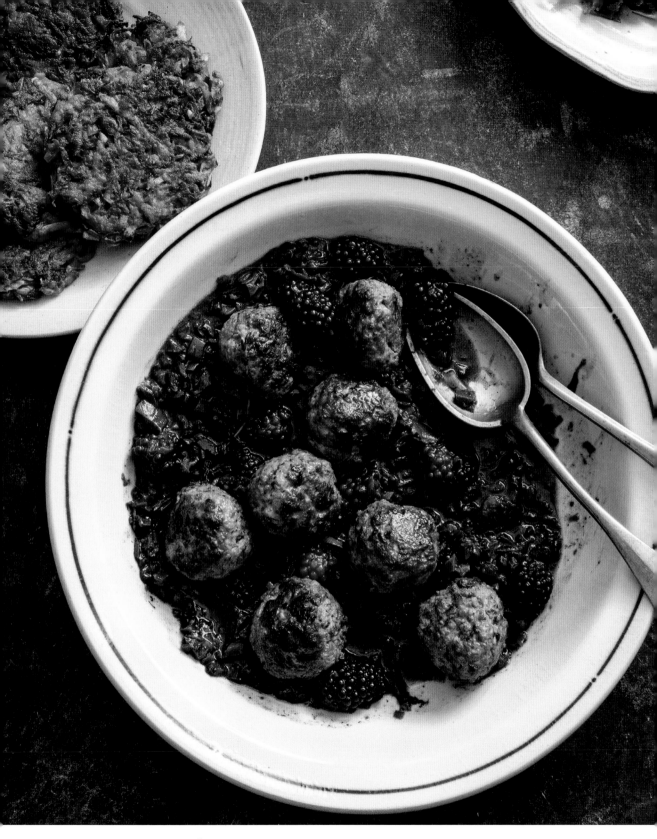

INFO PER SERVING (WITHOUT RÖSTI):   **PROTEIN** (G) 34.5   **CARBS** (G) 13   **SUGAR** (G) 7   **FAT** (G) 11   **SATURATED FAT** (G) 3.5

FIBRE (G) 4.5   **SALT** (G) 0.6

Serves: **4**

 Prep: **15 minutes**

 Cooking time: **about 50 minutes**

 Calories per serving with pasta/without pasta: **554/192**

BEEF OR VENISON RAGÙ WITH MUSHROOMS

1 tbsp olive oil

1 small onion, finely chopped

1 small carrot, finely chopped

1 celery stick, finely chopped

150g mushrooms (chestnut or portobellini), diced

300g lean minced beef or venison

3 garlic cloves, finely chopped

1 tsp mixed dried herbs

10g dried mushrooms, soaked in 100ml warm water

100ml red wine

100ml chopped tomatoes (canned are fine)

200ml beef or mushroom stock

100ml whole milk

freshly grated nutmeg

salt and black pepper

TO SERVE

400g flat pasta, such as pappardelle

Add this rich and flavourful ragù to a bowl of pasta and you'll have a supper fit for a king – or a Kingy! You might be surprised at the addition of milk but it is traditional in Italian-style meat sauce. It improves the texture and keeps the venison nice and moist.

Heat the oil in a saucepan or a flameproof casserole dish. Add the onion, carrot and celery and cook for several minutes until softened and lightly browned. Add the mushrooms and continue to cook until they have collapsed down. Add the beef or venison and the garlic and cook, stirring regularly, until the meat is well browned. Sprinkle in the herbs.

Drain the rehydrated mushrooms, reserving the soaking liquor, and chop finely. Add them to the pan and pour in the red wine. Bring to the boil and cook over a high heat until the wine has boiled off, then stir in the reserved mushroom liquor, the tomatoes and the stock. Season with salt and pepper.

Bring to the boil, then turn the heat down to a simmer. Partially cover the pan and leave to cook, stirring every so often, for half an hour. The sauce should look rich and be well reduced. Add the milk and continue to simmer for another few minutes. Taste for seasoning and adjust as necessary, then add a few rasps of nutmeg. Lovely served with pappardelle pasta.

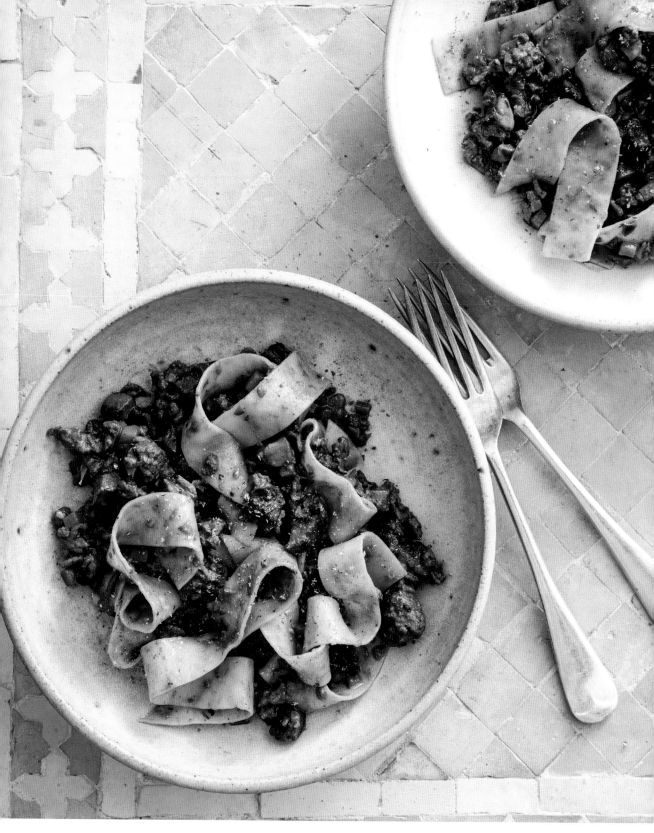

INFO PER SERVING WITH PASTA/WITHOUT PASTA: PROTEIN (G) 32/19   CARBS (G) 78/6   SUGAR (G) 7/5   FAT (G) 9/8

SATURATED FAT (G) 3/2.5   FIBRE (G) 7.5/3   SALT (G) 0.7/0.6

PUDD & BAI

BLUEBERRY CHEESECAKE
BRAMLEY APPLE SNOW
SPICED DATE & WALNUT LOAF
PEACH & RASPBERRY GALETTE
CHOCOLATE & RYE COOKIES
GREEN TEA & HONEY GRANITA

INGS
ES

TWO FRUITY COMPOTES
PEAR & GINGER CLAFOUTIS
COURGETTE & LIME CAKE
SWEET OMELETTES WITH BERRIES
CRUNCHY CHOCOLATE SLAB
LEMON & BUTTERMILK POSSET

Serves: **8**

 Prep: **15 minutes**

 Cooking time: **15 minutes, plus chilling time**

 Calories per slice: **219**

BLUEBERRY CHEESECAKE

100g granola (with no added sugar)

25g butter

150g cream cheese

125g buttermilk

1 tbsp honey

25g icing sugar

zest and juice of 1 lime

pinch of salt

200g blueberries

It's hard to make any sort of cheesecake entirely guilt-free, but we've done our best with this recipe – and it's a good one. Using granola that has no added sugar for the base helps to make this reasonably healthy and the buttermilk brings a lovely tangy taste to the topping. We've dropped the sugar as low as possible while keeping the flavour of the cake tip-top.

Line a deep 15cm-diameter cake tin with baking parchment. Preheat the oven to 180°C/Fan 160°C/Gas 4.

Put the granola into a food processor and blitz until it's well broken down. It doesn't have to be fine crumbs, though – it's good to have some texture. Melt the butter, add the granola and stir to combine, then press the mixture into the prepared tin. Bake for 15 minutes until the granola is lightly coloured, then remove from the oven and leave to cool.

Put the cream cheese into a bowl and beat until smooth. Add all the remaining ingredients, except the blueberries, and mix well. Sprinkle the blueberries over the granola base and pour the cream cheese mixture over the top. Smooth the mixture out as much as you can, then drop the tin on your work surface a couple of times to get rid of any air bubbles.

Leave the cheesecake in the fridge for several hours, or overnight, until set and well chilled before slicing and serving.

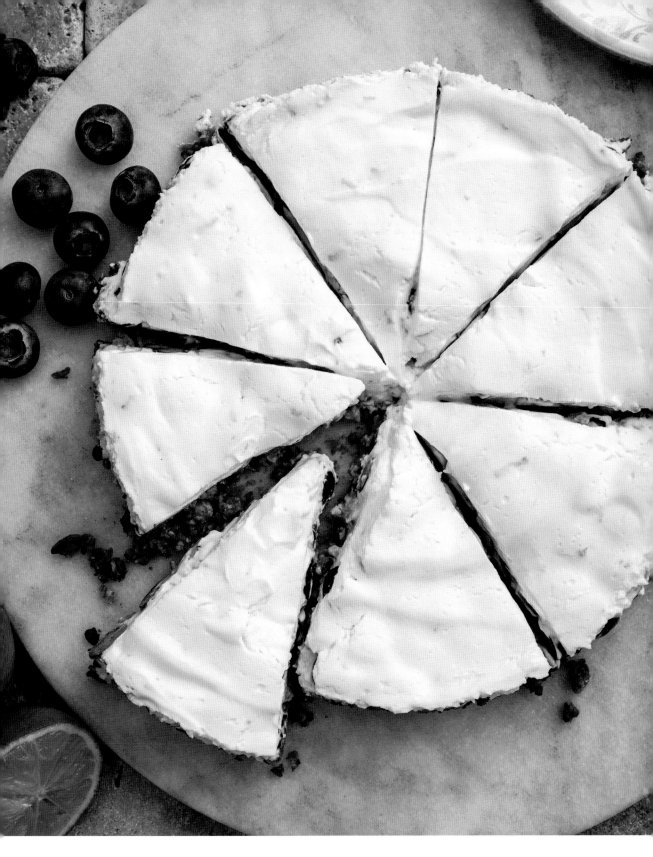

INFO PER SLICE: PROTEIN (G) 4   CARBS (G) 21   SUGAR (G) 13   FAT (G) 12.5   SATURATED FAT (G) 6.5   FIBRE (G) 3.5   SALT (G) 0.5

Serves: **4**

 Prep: **10 minutes**

 Cooking time:
about 15 minutes, plus chilling time

 Calories per serving:
126

500g (about 2 large) Bramley
    apples, peeled weight
juice of ½ lemon
1 cinnamon stick, broken up
2 egg whites
30g caster sugar

TO SERVE
25g amaretti biscuits
10g muscovado sugar
½ tsp ground cinnamon

BRAMLEY APPLE SNOW

Fun to make, apple snow is a good old traditional British pudding and one we both remember from our childhoods. For the sake of our waistlines we've cut down on the sugar in these quite a bit and no one has complained as yet.

Core and thinly slice the apples. Put them in a pan with the lemon juice, cinnamon stick and 75ml of water. Bring to the boil, then turn down the heat and cover the pan. Simmer, stirring every so often, until the apples soften into a purée – the slices will puff up and gently burst. This will take up to about 15 minutes.

Push the apples through a coarse sieve to remove any tough fibres, discarding the pieces of cinnamon stick as you go, then leave to cool to room temperature.

Whisk the egg whites to stiff peaks, then whisk in the sugar a teaspoon at a time, until the mixture has the consistency of meringue. Fold this into the apples and taste – add a little more sugar if you like, but the mixture should be quite tart. Divide between 4 bowls and chill in the fridge until cold – at least an hour.

Crumble up the amaretti biscuits and mix them with the sugar and cinnamon. Sprinkle them over the apple snow and serve.

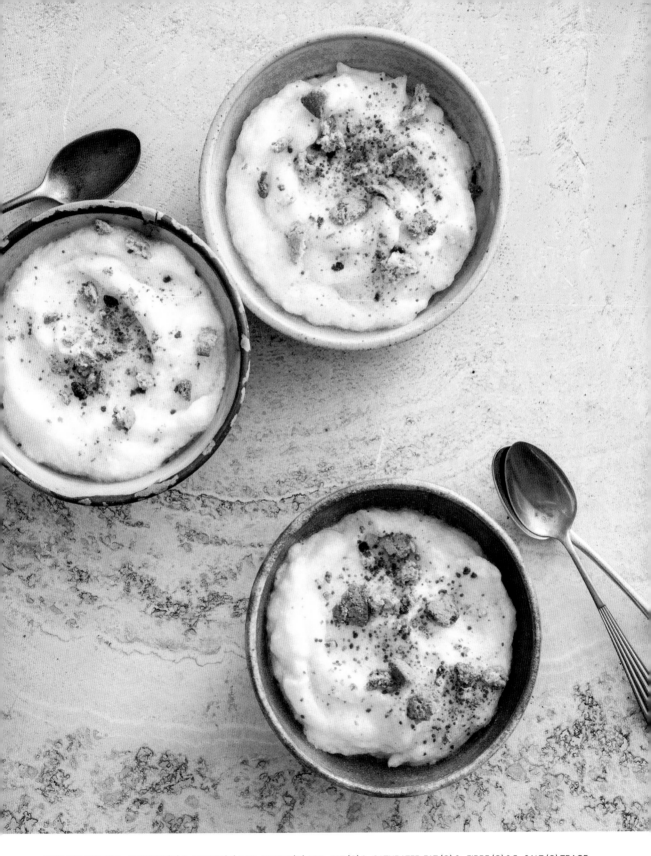

INFO PER SERVING: PROTEIN (G) 3   CARBS (G) 23.5   SUGAR (G) 23.5   FAT (G) 2   SATURATED FAT (G) 0   FIBRE (G) 2.5   SALT (G) TRACE

Makes: **12 slices**

 Prep: **15 minutes, plus standing time**

 Cooking time: **45–50 minutes**

 Calories per slice: **230**

SPICED DATE & WALNUT LOAF

225g wholemeal self-raising flour

1 tsp baking powder

¼ tsp ground cinnamon

¼ tsp ground cardamom

¼ tsp ground allspice

pinch of salt

100g butter

200g pitted dates, chopped

150ml freshly boiled water

pinch of saffron (optional)

50g maple syrup

50g light brown soft sugar

2 eggs

75g walnuts, roughly chopped

Packed full of spice and goodies, this is simple to make and just the ticket with a cuppa in the afternoon. Enjoy a slice just as it is or, if you're not counting the calories, spread with a little butter.

Preheat the oven to 180°C/Fan 160°C/Gas 4. Line a large (900g) loaf tin with some baking parchment.

Mix the flour with the baking powder and spices. Add a generous pinch of salt.

Put the butter and dates in a large bowl, cover with the boiled water and add the saffron, if using. Leave to stand for at least 20 minutes until the butter has melted and the dates have softened.

Stir in the maple syrup and sugar, then beat in the eggs. Fold in the flour and spice mixture, followed by the walnuts. Scrape the mixture into the prepared tin.

Bake in the oven for 45–50 minutes, until the top is springy and a skewer comes out clean. Leave the loaf to cool in the tin for 10 minutes before turning it out on to a rack to cool completely. Wrap the loaf in baking parchment and store in an airtight tin.

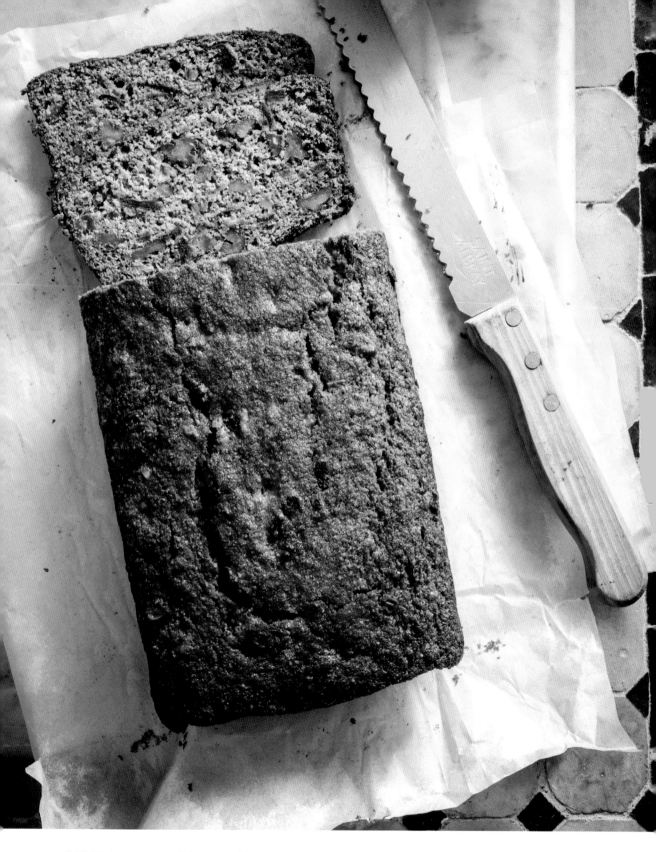

INFO PER SLICE: PROTEIN (G) 5   CARBS (G) 24   SUGAR (G) 12   FAT (G) 12   SATURATED FAT (G) 5   FIBRE (G) 1   SALT (G) 0.6

Serves: **6**

 Prep: **20 minutes, plus chilling time**

 Cooking time: **about 25–30 minutes**

 Calories per serving: **352**

PEACH & RASPBERRY GALETTE

PASTRY
175g wholemeal plain flour
75g ground almonds
pinch of salt
50g butter, chilled and diced
1 egg
100ml Greek yoghurt

FILLING
2 tbsp ground almonds
1 tbsp light brown soft sugar
3 ripe peaches, cut into
    wedges (or canned
    peaches)
200g raspberries

Galette can mean different things – a Breton galette is a type of pancake – but this one is a free-form, open-topped pie. We've made a special pastry that swaps some of the butter for yoghurt to make it a bit healthier; hope you like it. You could use any fruit, but peaches and raspberries are a marriage made in heaven.

First make the pastry. Put the flour and ground almonds into a bowl and add a generous pinch of salt. Add the butter and rub it in until the mixture resembles breadcrumbs. Beat the egg and reserve 1 tablespoon of it. Mix the remaining egg with the yoghurt and add it to the bowl. Cut the mixture with a knife until it starts to form clumps, then bring everything together into a smooth dough with your hands. Wrap the pastry and chill it in the fridge for at least an hour.

Preheat the oven to 200°C/Fan 180°C/Gas 6. Line a large baking tray with some greaseproof paper.

Roll out the pastry into a large round that's about ½cm thick and place it on the baking tray. Mix the 2 tablespoons of ground almonds and half the sugar together and sprinkle over the centre of the pastry, leaving a 3–4cm border all the way around. Arrange the fruit on top, then sprinkle with the rest of the sugar. Fold in the uncovered edges of pastry so they cover some of the filling, leaving the centre exposed.

Mix the reserved tablespoon of egg with 1–2 teaspoons of water and brush this over the pastry. Bake the galette in the preheated oven for 25–30 minutes, until the pastry is crisp and golden brown and the fruit has softened. Serve warm or cold.

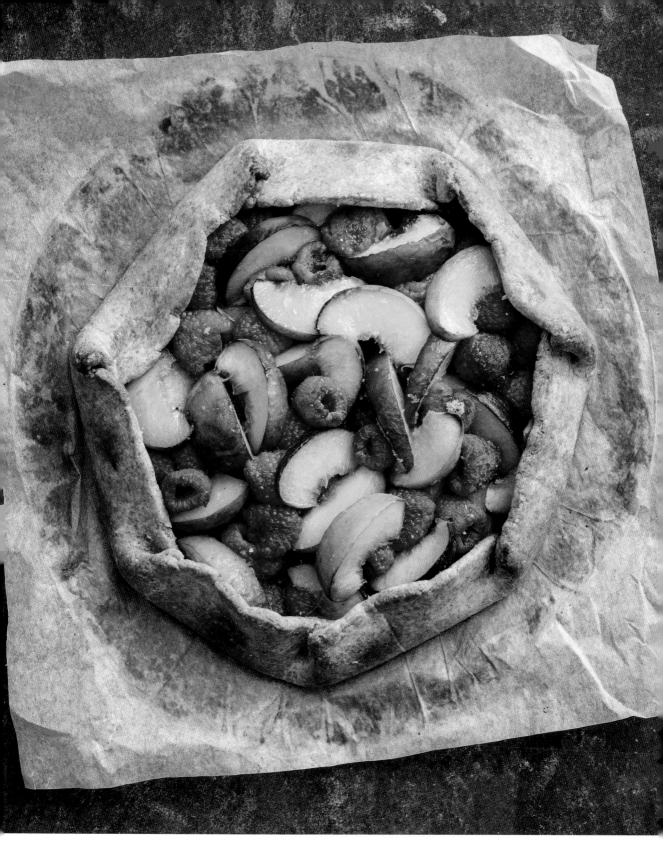

INFO PER SERVING: PROTEIN (G) 11   CARBS (G) 29   SUGAR (G) 10   FAT (G) 20   SATURATED FAT (G) 6.5   FIBRE (G) 5   SALT (G) 0.4

Makes: **16**

 Prep: **20 minutes, plus chilling time**

 Cooking time: **10–12 minutes**

 Calories per cookie: **114**

35g rye flour

15g cocoa powder

½ tsp bicarbonate of soda

pinch of salt

150g dark chocolate

50g butter, diced

½ tsp vanilla extract

2 eggs

85g soft light brown sugar

CHOCOLATE & RYE COOKIES

In fact, these little lovelies are more like mini chocolate cakes than cookies, as they're quite fudgy with crispy edges and worryingly delicious. It's hard to eat just one. They're very soft when they first come out of the oven, but don't be tempted to leave them for longer, as they get overcooked very quickly. Leave them to cool and harden before eating and your patience will be rewarded.

Put the flour, cocoa and bicarbonate of soda in a bowl with a generous pinch of salt and mix thoroughly. Set aside.

Break up the chocolate and put it in a heatproof bowl with the butter. Set the bowl over a pan of simmering water and stir the chocolate and butter regularly until they are completely melted and well combined. Add the vanilla extract and remove the bowl from the heat. Leave to cool for about 10 minutes.

Put the eggs and sugar in a bowl, or in a stand mixer, and beat until the mixture is well aerated and mousse-like – you should be able to trail a ribbon with the beater by the time it is done. This will take at least 5 minutes.

Pour the chocolate and butter mixture into the eggs, then gently fold everything together until it is dark and streak free. Fold in the flour mixture. The batter will still be very wet, but don't worry, it will firm up in the fridge. Put the bowl in the fridge and leave the mixture to chill for at least half an hour.

Preheat the oven to 180°C/Fan 160°C/Gas 4 and line 2 baking trays with baking parchment. Using a wet spoon, spoon the mixture into about 16 portions, spacing them out well as they will spread a lot. Wet your hands and shape each one into a ball, then flatten them slightly.

Bake in the preheated oven for 10–12 minutes, until the cookies have spread and started to crack on top. Remove them from the oven and leave to cool on the baking trays. Store in an airtight tin.

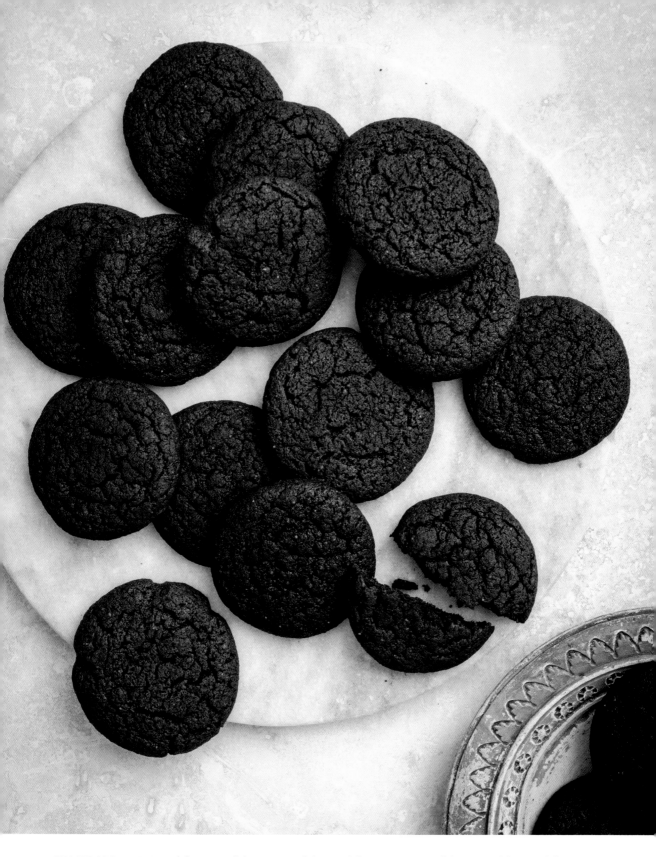

INFO PER COOKIE: PROTEIN (G) 2   CARBS (G) 12.5   SUGAR (G) 11   FAT (G) 6   SATURATED FAT (G) 3.5   FIBRE (G) 1   SALT (G) 0.3

Serves: **4**

 Prep: **10 minutes, plus freezing time**

 Cooking time:
no cooking

 Calories per serving: **62**

85g honey

a few mint sprigs, plus extra to garnish

zest and juice of 1 lemon

2 green tea or matcha tea bags

GREEN TEA & HONEY GRANITA

Dairy-free and low in calories, granita is a real Sicilian summer treat. This frozen dessert is usually made with fruit juice but our refreshing honey and green tea or matcha version is a real winner.

Bring a kettle of water to the boil and leave to stand for a minute. Put the honey, mint, lemon zest and lemon juice into a saucepan. Pour over 750ml of the just-boiled water and stir until the honey has dissolved. Add the tea bags.

Leave to steep for 5 minutes, then remove the tea bags and discard them. Leave the mixture to cool to room temperature, then strain it through a sieve into a fairly shallow freezer container.

Freeze the mixture for at least half an hour until it has started to set around the edges. Break up the frozen bits and work into the less solid middle, then freeze again. Repeat this every half hour until the granita has frozen into crystals.

Remove the granita from the freezer 10 minutes before you want to serve it. Break it up with a fork and spoon into glasses. Garnish with a few fresh mint sprigs.

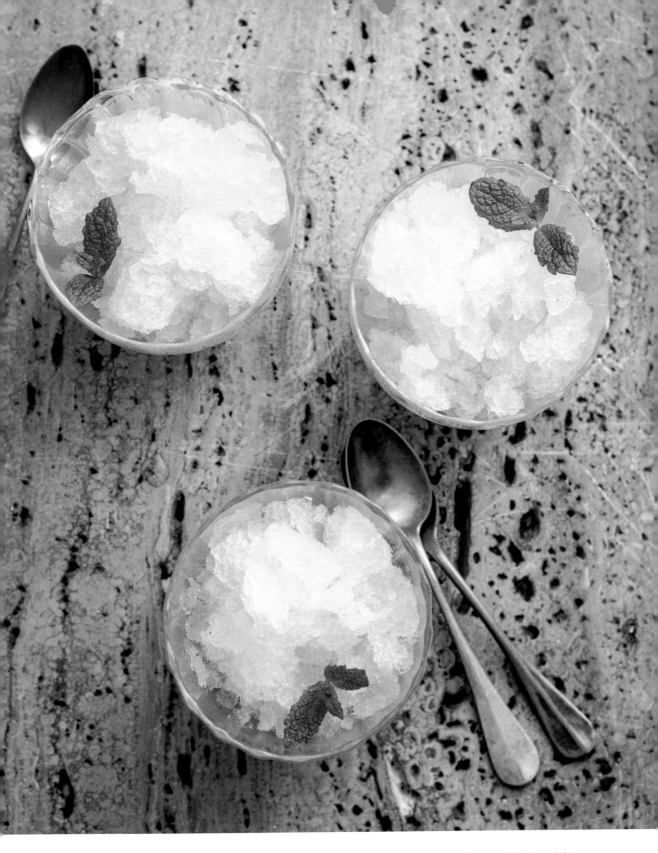

INFO PER SERVING: PROTEIN (G) 0   CARBS (G) 15.5   SUGAR (G) 15.5   FAT (G) 0   SATURATED FAT (G) 0   FIBRE (G) 0   SALT (G) 0

Serves: **4**

Prep: **5–10 minutes**

Cooking time:
10–20 minutes

Calories per serving:
Dried apricot: **168**
Plum & blackberry: **61**

TWO FRUITY COMPOTES

DRIED APRICOT COMPOTE

250g dried apricots (the soft orange
   ones work well)
2 tbsp honey
juice of 1 orange
1 tsp cardamom pods

1 piece of cinnamon stick
2 pieces of pared lemon zest
a few drops of rosewater
   (optional)

Put the apricots in a small pan and drizzle over the honey. Add all the remaining ingredients and just enough water to cover the apricots. Stir over a low heat until the honey has dissolved, then turn up the heat and bring it to the boil. Turn down to a simmer again and cover. Cook for 15–20 minutes, stirring regularly, until the apricots are tender, then add the rosewater, if using. Leave the apricots to cool in the liquid, then transfer everything to a container, removing the cinnamon stick, and store in the fridge. Both these compotes are great with your breakfast granola or just with some yoghurt for a speedy pudding.

PLUM & BLACKBERRY COMPOTE

6 plums, pitted and roughly chopped
1 tbsp light brown soft sugar
2 bay leaves

a few peppercorns, lightly cracked
juice of ½ lemon
150g blackberries

This is a good recipe for using up any plums that aren't quite nice enough to eat raw and need a bit of TLC.

Put the plums in a saucepan and sprinkle over the sugar. Add the bay leaves and peppercorns and pour over the lemon juice and 50ml of water. Stir until the sugar has dissolved, then cover and leave to cook gently until the plums have softened. This will take anything between 5 and 10 minutes, depending on the ripeness of the plums. Add the blackberries and cook for a further minute or so until the blackberries start releasing their juice, then remove from the heat. The compote will thicken as it cools. Transfer to a container and store in the fridge.

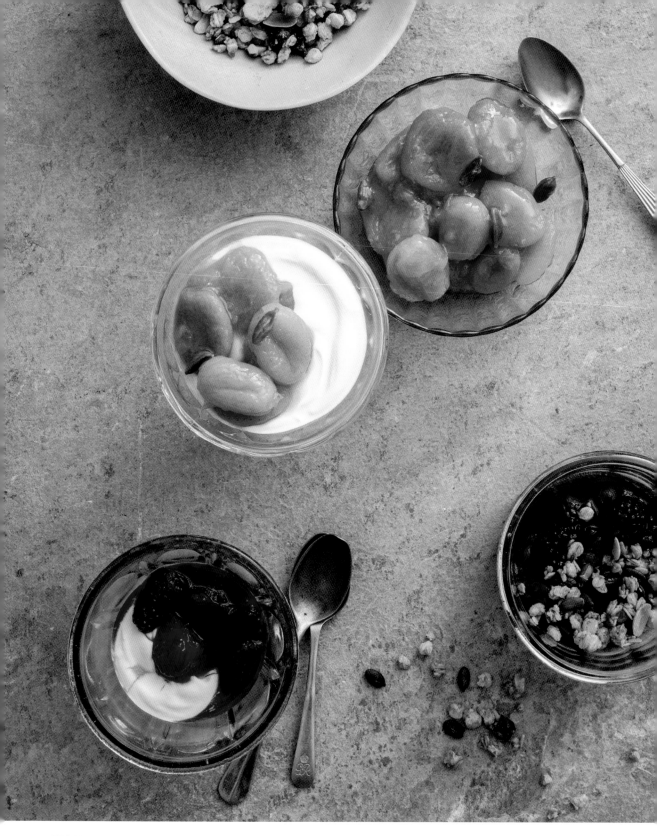

INFO PER SERVING OF COMPOTE – DRIED APRICOT/PLUM & BLACKBERRY: PROTEIN (G) 3/1 CARBS (G) 35/12 SUGAR (G) 35/12

FAT (G) 0/0 SATURATED FAT (G) 0/0 FIBRE (G) 6/3 SALT (G) 0/0

Serves: **4**

 Prep: **10 minutes**

 Cooking time:
25–30 minutes

 Calories per serving:
398

PEAR & GINGER CLAFOUTIS

5g butter

1 tbsp ground almonds

2 tbsp light brown soft sugar

1 tsp ground ginger

2 ripe pears, peeled and cut
　　into slim wedges

BATTER

50g ground almonds

25g plain flour

40g caster sugar

pinch of salt

2 eggs

200ml whole milk

50ml crème fraiche or yoghurt

2 tbsp flaked almonds

TO SERVE

crème fraiche (optional)

A clafoutis is a popular French dessert of fruit baked in a batter and very good it is too. The traditional version is made with cherries, but we think pears work just as well. Ideally the pears need to be nice and ripe, but you could always used tinned pears instead.

Preheat the oven to 180°C/Fan 160°C/Gas 4. First prepare the dish. Rub the butter over a shallow ovenproof dish. Mix the tablespoon of ground almonds with a tablespoon of the sugar and ½ teaspoon of ground ginger and sprinkle this over the buttered dish.

Toss the pears in the remaining brown sugar and ginger and arrange them over the base of the dish.

For the batter, put the ground almonds, flour and caster sugar into a bowl and add a generous pinch of salt. Whisk in the eggs, then add the milk and crème fraiche or yoghurt. Pour the batter into the oven dish around the pears, then sprinkle the flaked almonds over the top.

Bake in the oven for 25–30 minutes until the batter and almonds are a light golden brown and the batter has puffed up a little. Serve with crème fraiche, if you like.

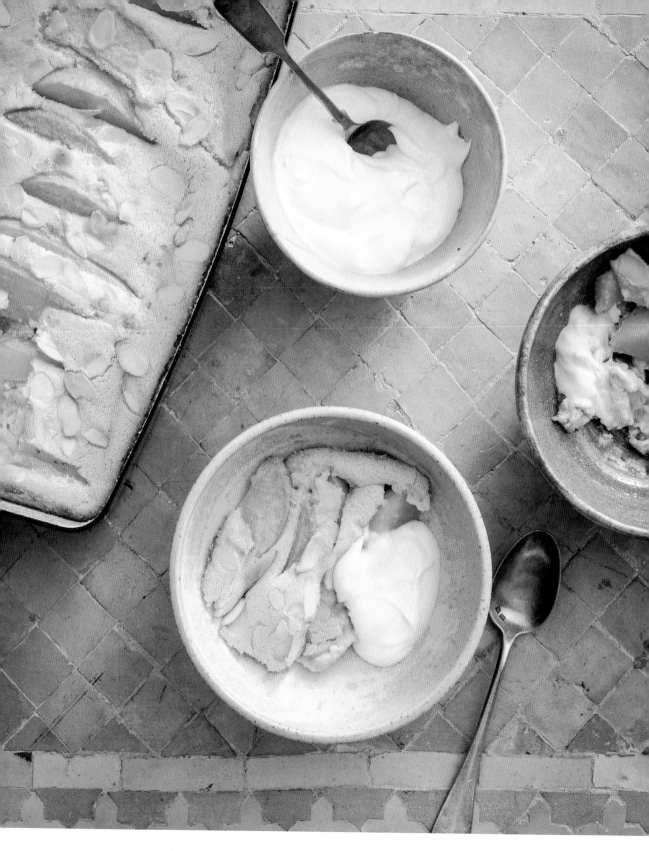

INFO PER SERVING: PROTEIN (G) 13   CARBS (G) 32   SUGAR (G) 27   FAT (G) 24   SATURATED FAT (G) 7   FIBRE (G) 2   SALT (G) 0.5

Makes: **12 slices**

 Prep: **20 minutes**

 Cooking time:
about 30 minutes

 Calories per slice: **271**

COURGETTE & LIME CAKE

300g courgettes, coarsely
   grated
125g plain flour (preferably
   wholemeal)
125g ground almonds
1 tsp baking powder
½ tsp bicarbonate of soda
pinch of salt
100g caster sugar
2 eggs
75g olive oil
75g plain yoghurt
zest and juice of 2 limes

TOPPING (OPTIONAL)
200g cream cheese
3 tbsp icing sugar
zest of 1 lime, plus extra
   to garnish
juice of ½ a lime

We love that we can get some of our five-a-day in cake form! Courgettes make a lovely moist cake and the lime really lifts the flavour to another level. Try this and we're sure you'll love it. If you don't fancy the cream cheese icing, simply dust the cake with icing sugar and serve with some very slightly sweetened crème fraiche.

Preheat the oven to 200°C/Fan 180°C/Gas 6. Line a deep 20cm-diameter cake tin with baking parchment.

Sprinkle the courgettes into a clean tea towel and twist into a bundle. Squeeze well to get rid of all the excess liquid in the courgettes.

Put the flour, ground almonds, baking powder and bicarbonate of soda into a bowl and add a generous pinch of salt.

Whisk together the sugar, eggs and olive oil until well combined. Add the yoghurt, then the lime zest and juice – the mixture may curdle slightly, but don't worry, it won't affect the end result. Add the squeezed courgettes, then fold in the dry ingredients.

Scrape the mixture into the prepared tin and bake the cake in the oven for about 30 minutes, until well risen and golden brown. Remove from the oven and leave the cake to cool in the tin for 10 minutes, then transfer it to a cooling rack.

For the optional topping, put the cream cheese in a bowl and beat to break it up. Beat in the sugar, lime zest and juice. Using a palette knife, swirl the mixture over the cake, then put it in the fridge to firm up. Sprinkle with extra lime zest before serving.

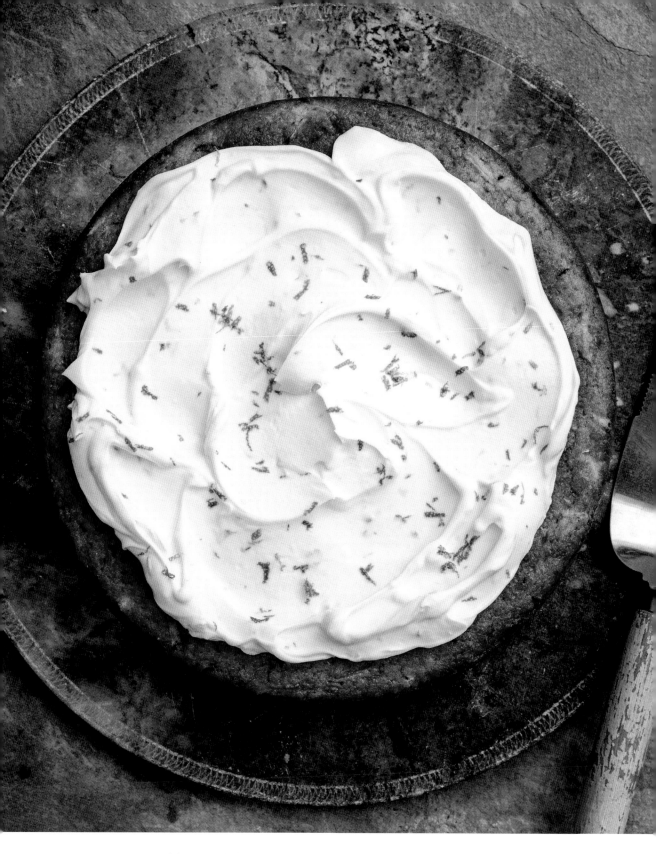

INFO PER SLICE: PROTEIN (G) 7   CARBS (G) 22.5   SUGAR (G) 14   FAT (G) 17   SATURATED FAT (G) 4   FIBRE (G) 1   SALT (G) 0.5

Serves: **4**

 Prep: **5 minutes**

 Cooking time:
about 20 minutes

 Calories per serving:
262

SWEET OMELETTES WITH BERRIES

BERRIES
500g frozen mixed berries
juice of ½ lemon
1 tbsp caster sugar or honey

OMELETTES
8 eggs
4 tsp sugar
½ tsp cinnamon
4 tsp butter
salt

TO SERVE (OPTIONAL)
crème fraiche or yoghurt

No reason why omelettes should always be savoury. A sweet omelette makes a really nice quick dessert, especially when partnered with a fruity compote. Those packs of frozen berries you find in the supermarket containing a mix of strawberries, raspberries, blackberries, redcurrants and blackcurrants are just the job for this recipe, so you can make it at any time of year.

Put the berries into a saucepan and add the lemon juice and the sugar or honey. Stir over a low heat until the sugar or honey has dissolved, then cover the pan and leave the fruit to cook very gently until it has all defrosted. You will find that the fruit will release enough juice to create a sauce without having to add any extra liquid. Leave the pan of fruit over a low heat while you make the omelettes.

Make each omelette individually. Beat 2 eggs and add a pinch of salt, a teaspoon of sugar and a pinch of cinnamon. Heat an omelette pan and add a teaspoon of butter. Swirl it around and as soon as it has melted and started foaming, pour in the eggs and swirl to cover the base of the pan. Using a fork, pull in the edges as they set, allowing any uncooked egg to fill the space, until the omelette is just about set.

Transfer the omelette to a plate, ladle some of the compote on to one side of the omelette, then fold the other side over. Repeat with the remaining omelette ingredients. Serve with dollops of crème fraiche or yoghurt, if using.

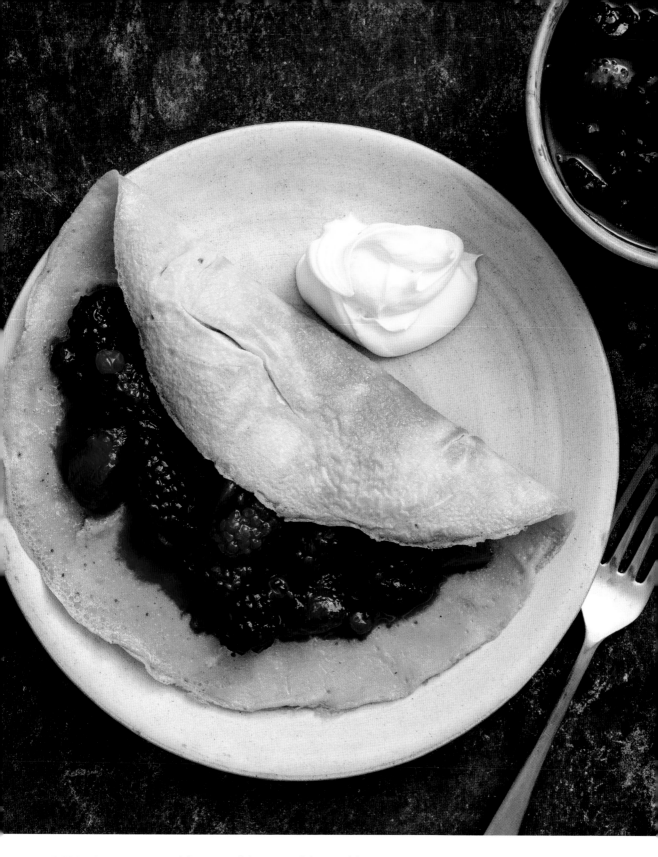

INFO PER SERVING: PROTEIN (G) 17 CARBS (G) 13 SUGAR (G) 13 FAT (G) 15 SATURATED FAT (G) 6 FIBRE (G) 3 SALT (G) 0.6

Serves: **10–12**

 Prep: **10 minutes**

 Cooking time:
5 minutes, plus chilling

 Calories per 25g: **131**

CRUNCHY CHOCOLATE SLAB

vegetable oil, for greasing

75g coconut oil

50g cocoa powder

50g runny honey

a few drops of vanilla extract

pinch of salt

50g raisins or sultanas, or
    chopped prunes, dates
    or figs

25g nuts, roughly chopped
    (we used pistachios)

25g mixed seeds

This is a sort of home-made chocolate bar that you can tailor to your own taste and desires. We've added dried fruit, nuts and seeds, but you can add whatever you fancy. It would be banging with spices like ginger, cardamom and cinnamon, if they're your thing. Coconut oil can soften at room temperature, so it's best to keep this slab of deliciousness in the fridge.

Lightly oil a dish measuring 12–15cm by 18–20cm, then line it with cling film or greaseproof paper.

Melt the coconut oil in a small saucepan, then stir in the cocoa powder, honey and vanilla extract. Add a pinch of salt, then whisk to combine and get rid of any lumps of cocoa powder.

Pour the mixture into the prepared dish, then sprinkle over the dried fruit, followed by the nuts and then the seeds. You'll find that the dried fruit sinks, while most of the nuts remain visible just below the surface and the seeds provide a coating.

Transfer the dish to the fridge and leave the mixture to set for several hours until completely solid. Cut the chocolate into pieces with a sharp knife (or just break it up), then store it in the fridge in an airtight container.

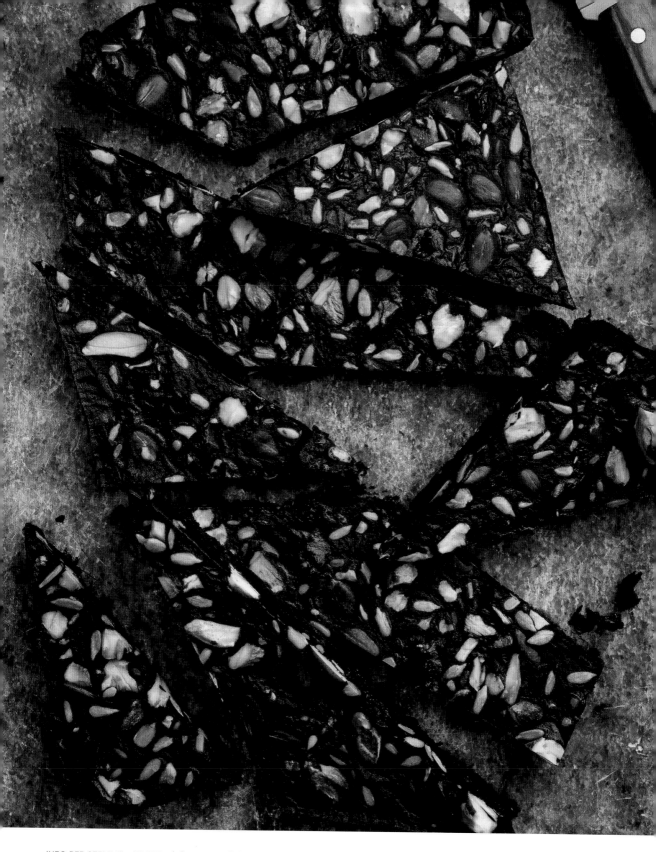

INFO PER SERVING: PROTEIN (G) 2 CARBS (G) 7 SUGAR (G) 6.5 FAT (G) 10 SATURATED FAT (G) 7 FIBRE (G) 1 SALT (G) TRACE

Serves: **4**

 Prep: **5 minutes**

 Cooking time:
**about 5 minutes, plus
chilling time**

 Calories per serving:
316

200ml double cream

50g caster sugar

pared zest and juice of 1 lemon

200ml buttermilk

TO SERVE
grated lemon zest

biscuits (optional)

LEMON &
BUTTERMILK
POSSET

A posset is a delightful little pud that's basically just a thickened cream flavoured with lemon. Here we make it with half cream and half buttermilk which adds a nice tangy flavour. This is a great one to prepare in advance and have ready in the fridge – and it's even better served with a crisp biscuit if you have some.

Put the cream in a small saucepan with the caster sugar and the lemon zest. Heat gently, stirring until the sugar has dissolved, then bring the mixture to the boil. Simmer for 3 minutes, then remove the pan from the heat.

Pour the lemon juice and buttermilk into a bowl and whisk to combine. Strain the double cream mixture into a jug, then pour this from a height over the lemon and buttermilk, whisking as you do so. When the cream and buttermilk are combined, pour the mixture into 4 glasses or bowls.

Chill in the fridge for at least an hour – the mixture thickens almost immediately but the possets are best served cold. Serve, sprinkled with a little grated lemon zest.

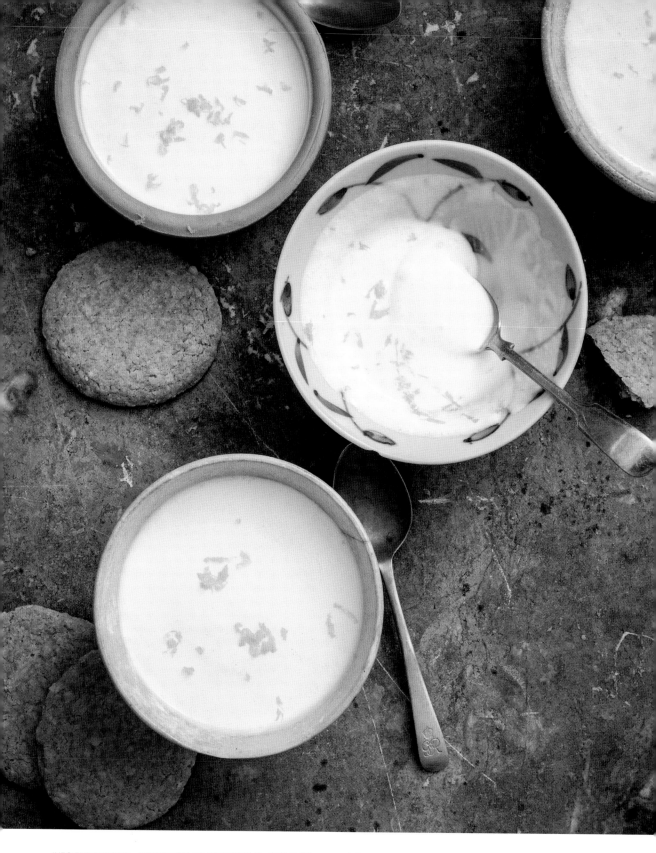

INFO PER SERVING: PROTEIN (G) 2.5 CARBS (G) 16 SUGAR (G) 16 FAT (G) 27 SATURATED FAT (G) 17 FIBRE (G) 0 SALT (G) 0.1

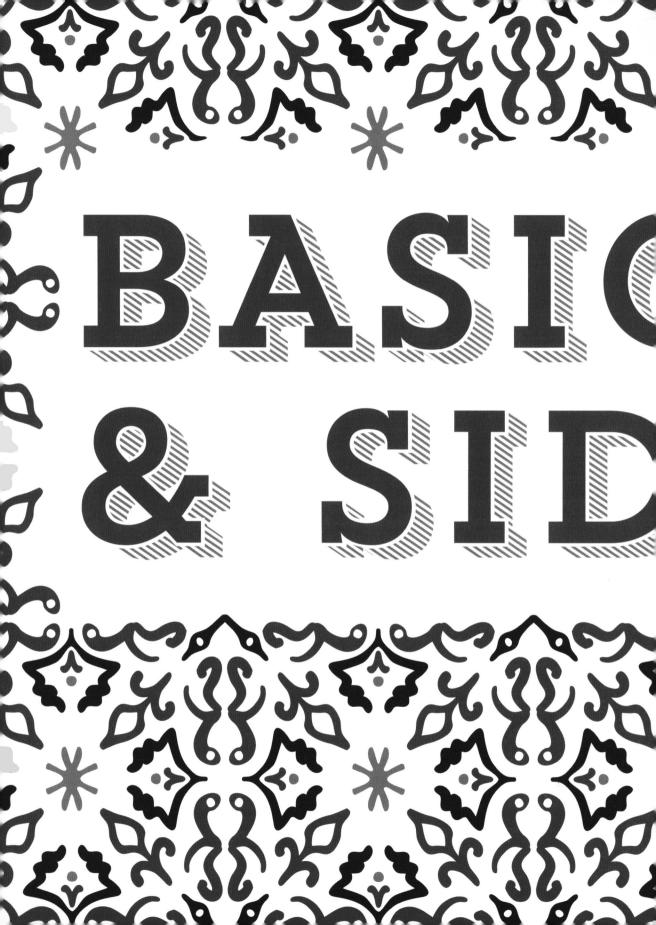

BASIC
& SID

SES

- THREE-ROOT RÖSTI
- GRIDDLED SPROUTING BROCCOLI
- SLOW-COOKED GREEN BEANS
- BEETROOT & WALNUT SALAD
- BRAISED BUCKWHEAT
- WHOLEGRAIN RICE PILAF
- COURGETTE SALAD
- VEGETABLE STOCK
- CHICKEN STOCK

Serves: **4**

 Prep: **15 minutes, plus standing time**

Cooking time: **about 12 minutes**

Calories per serving: **323**

THREE-ROOT RÖSTI

150g beetroot, coarsely grated

150g carrots, coarsely grated

200g potatoes, coarsely grated

1 onion, finely chopped

2 garlic cloves, grated or crushed

1 egg, beaten

25g plain flour

1 tsp mustard powder

1 tsp dried thyme or mixed herbs

4 tbsp olive oil

salt and black pepper

Rösti are usually made with just potatoes but you can use any other root veg too. Here we are using a mix of beetroot, carrot and potatoes but celeriac and parsnips would also work well. These make a brilliant accompaniment to meat or fish dishes or they're great on their own as a tasty little snack.

Put the vegetables in a colander and sprinkle them with salt. Leave to stand for half an hour, then wrap them in a clean tea towel and gently squeeze to remove any liquid that hasn't already drained away.

Put the vegetables in a bowl with the garlic. Stir in the egg, flour, mustard powder and herbs, then add a little more salt and some pepper. Stir thoroughly to combine. The mixture should be slightly sticky, but if it feels a bit too wet, add a little more flour.

Form the mixture into 8 patties, pressing them firmly so everything sticks together. Heat half the oil in a large frying pan and add 4 of the patties. Fry over a medium heat for several minutes on each side until crisp and golden – be careful not to flip them for the first time until you know a decent crust has developed as they are liable to break up if not cooked enough.

Keep warm and add the remaining olive oil to the pan to cook the rest of the rösti.

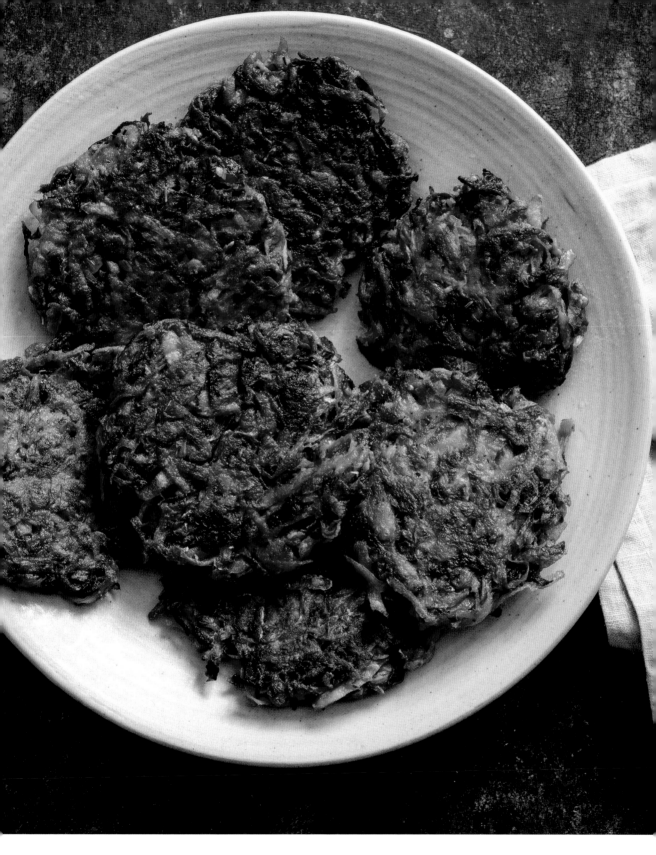

INFO PER SERVING: PROTEIN (G) 5   CARBS (G) 20.5   SUGAR (G) 5.5   FAT (G) 13   SATURATED FAT (G) 2   FIBRE (G) 5   SALT (G) 0.2

Serves: **4**

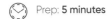 Prep: **5 minutes**

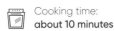 Cooking time:
about 10 minutes

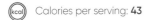 Calories per serving: **43**

GRIDDLED SPROUTING BROCCOLI

400g sprouting broccoli,
    trimmed
squeeze of lemon juice
salt and black pepper

This is a good way to cook broccoli – it grills and steams at the same time and is really tasty. No oil needed and you don't have to blanch the broccoli first. If you do fancy a bit of oil, just toss the broccoli in a tablespoon of olive oil before putting it on the griddle.

Heat a griddle pan until it's too hot to hold your hand over for more than a few seconds. Add the broccoli spears and turn the heat down slightly. Leave them to cook for a minute, then turn and cook for another minute.

At this point, splash a tablespoon of water over the pan – it will hiss and sizzle and create steam around the broccoli. Keep cooking the broccoli, turning it every 30 seconds or so and adding a little more water each time you turn, until it is just cooked through and lightly charred. This should take about 7–8 minutes.

Remove the broccoli from the griddle and season with salt and pepper. Squeeze over some lemon juice before serving.

INFO PER SERVING (NO OIL): PROTEIN (G) 4   CARBS (G) 3   SUGAR (G) 2   FAT (G) 0   SATURATED FAT (G) 0   FIBRE (G) 4   SALT (G) TRACE

Serves: **4**

 Prep: **10 minutes**

 Cooking time:
about 30 minutes

 Calories per 100g: **50**

2 tbsp olive oil
1 onion, finely chopped
3 garlic cloves, finely chopped
500g green beans, trimmed
2 large tomatoes (about 300g),
    finely chopped or puréed
1 tsp dried oregano
100ml white wine
salt and black pepper

SLOW-COOKED GREEN BEANS

This is a very popular side dish in Italy and a lovely thing to have in the fridge to partner meat, fish or almost anything. It keeps well for a few days. You could use canned tomatoes, but we reckon fresh are the best thing here.

Heat the olive oil in a large flameproof casserole dish or a lidded sauté pan. Add the onion and sauté until soft and translucent. Add the garlic and cook for a further couple of minutes, then stir in the beans and tomatoes. Season with salt and pepper and sprinkle in the oregano.

Pour the white wine into the pan and bring to the boil. Turn down the heat and cover the pan. Cook slowly for up to half an hour, stirring every so often, until the tomatoes have completely broken down and the beans are very tender.

Good hot, cold or at room temperature.

INFO PER 100G: PROTEIN (G) 1 CARBS (G) 3.5 SUGAR (G) 3 FAT (G) 2.3 SATURATED FAT (G) 0.5 FIBRE (G) 2 SALT (G) TRACE

Serves: **4**

 Prep: **10 minutes**

 Cooking time:
**30 minutes or more,
depending on size**

 Calories per serving:
179

BEETROOT & WALNUT SALAD

500g whole beetroots,
    preferably medium sized and
    with their leaves
3 tbsp olive oil
2 garlic cloves, finely chopped
1 tbsp red wine vinegar
2 tbsp walnuts, chopped and
    lightly toasted
salt and black pepper

If you can buy a lovely bunch of beetroot with the leaves fresh and intact all the better, as you can use the leaves in the salad. Beetroots are packed with valuable nutrients so super-good for you as well as being totally delicious. This makes a perfect accompaniment to meat or fish or you could serve it as a little starter, perhaps with some goat's cheese crumbled over the top.

If using bunched beetroots, twist or cut off the beetroots from the stems, about 2cm away from the beetroot head. Pick over the leaves and keep any worth cooking.

Put the unpeeled beetroots into a saucepan, cover with freshly boiled water and add salt. Bring to the boil and simmer until tender. Small beetroots will take about 20 minutes to be knife tender, but very large ones may take up to an hour. Start testing medium-sized beetroots for doneness after about 25 minutes.

When the beetroots are cooked through, drain and cool them with cold water. Rub off the skins and slice the beets into ½cm rounds.

If you are using the leaves, wash them thoroughly and put them in a pan with a splash of water. Cook until they have just wilted, then remove from the pan and drain.

Heat the olive oil in a small frying pan. Add the garlic and cook it very gently just to take the raw edge off the flavour and infuse the oil. Add the red wine vinegar and swirl it around the pan, then remove the pan from the heat.

Arrange the beetroot slices and leaves, if using, in a shallow serving dish, then season with salt and pepper. Drizzle over the garlic oil, then sprinkle with the walnuts.

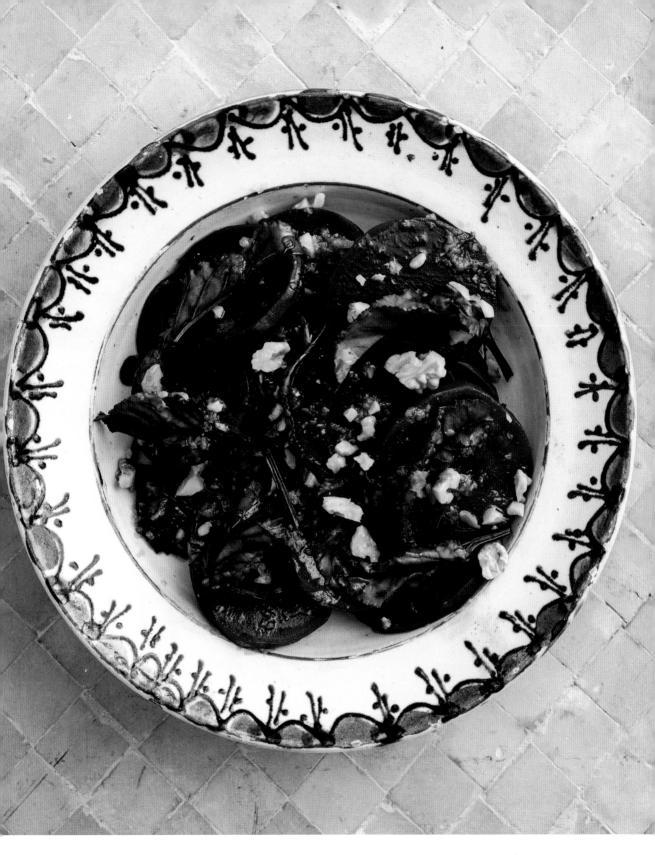

INFO PER SERVING: PROTEIN (G) 3.5   CARBS (G) 9.5   SUGAR (G) 8.5   FAT (G) 13.5   SATURATED FAT (G) 2   FIBRE (G) 3.5   SALT (G) 0.2

Serves: **4**

 Prep: **5 minutes**

 Cooking time:
20–30 minutes

 Calories per serving:
240

BRAISED BUCKWHEAT

1 tbsp olive oil

1 onion, finely chopped

2 garlic cloves, finely chopped

200g buckwheat groats, rinsed

1 thyme sprig or ½ tsp dried thyme

½ tsp ground allspice

400ml vegetable or mushroom stock

parsley or dill, to garnish

salt and black pepper

Buckwheat makes a great alternative to rice and is rich in fibre and antioxidants, so is a healthy choice. Despite its name, buckwheat is not a type of wheat and is gluten free.

Heat the olive oil in a saucepan and add the onion. Sauté until soft and translucent, then add the garlic and buckwheat. Stir to toast the buckwheat for a couple of minutes, then stir in the thyme and allspice. Season with salt and pepper.

Pour in the stock and bring to the boil, then turn the heat down to a simmer and cover the pan. Simmer for about 20 minutes until all the liquid has been absorbed and the buckwheat groats are cooked through but still have a bit of bite. Leave to stand for another 10 minutes before serving. Nice garnished with parsley or dill.

INFO PER SERVING: PROTEIN (G) 6.5   CARBS (G) 44   SUGAR (G) 2.5   FAT (G) 4   SATURATED FAT (G) 0.5   FIBRE (G) 3   SALT (G) 0.65

Serves: **4**

 Prep: **10 minutes**

 Cooking time:
20–30 minutes

 Calories per serving:
325

WHOLEGRAIN RICE PILAF

1 tbsp olive or coconut oil

1 onion, finely chopped

5g root ginger, finely chopped

2 garlic cloves, finely chopped

1 bay leaf

250g wholegrain rice of your choice

1 medium tomato, finely chopped

400ml vegetable or chicken stock or water

1 small bunch of parsley or coriander, finely chopped

leaves from a small bunch of mint, finely chopped

2 tbsp flaked almonds, lightly toasted (optional)

2 spring onions, finely sliced on the diagonal

salt and black pepper

This is a lovely herby pilaf that is a great accompaniment to meat, fish or veggie dishes. You can use wild, black or red rice or brown basmati. Brown basmati usually takes about 20 minutes to cook, red rice 22–25 minutes and black rice up to 30 minutes.

Heat the oil in a saucepan, then add the onion and sauté until soft and translucent. Stir in the ginger, garlic and bay leaf, followed by the rice and tomato. Stir for a couple of minutes and season with salt and pepper.

Pour in the stock or water. Bring to the boil, then cover the pan, reduce the heat and simmer for 20–30 minutes, depending on which rice you're using. When the rice is the soft side of al dente and the liquid has been absorbed, remove the pan from the heat, place a tea towel over it and put the lid on top. Leave to stand for 10 minutes.

Stir in the herbs, then garnish with the toasted almonds, if using, and the spring onions.

INFO PER SERVING: PROTEIN (G) 9   CARBS (G) 51   SUGAR (G) 4.5   FAT (G) 8   SATURATED FAT (G) 1   FIBRE (G) 4   SALT (G) 0.6

Serves: **4**

 Prep: **5 minutes**

 Cooking time:
no cooking

 Calories: **95**

COURGETTE SALAD

2 medium courgettes, cut into ribbons

2 tbsp olive oil

zest and juice of ½ lemon

2 tsp white balsamic vinegar (can use dark if necessary)

a few thyme or lemon thyme leaves

a few basil leaves, torn

25g Parmesan cheese or similar

salt and black pepper

Slender courgette ribbons make a very pretty salad. If you have one of those spiralisers everyone bought a while back, use that to make the ribbons, but if yours, like ours, has broken, try a y-shaped peeler or a mandolin. Be sure only to season this salad just before serving, as the salt will make the courgettes release liquid.

First blot the courgette ribbons between a couple of clean tea towels or some kitchen paper. Unless the courgettes are very small they will release a lot of liquid.

Arrange the courgette ribbons in a shallow serving bowl. Whisk the olive oil, lemon zest and juice and balsamic vinegar together. Drizzle this over the courgettes, turning them over very gently so they are lightly coated.

Just before serving, season with salt and pepper and sprinkle over the herbs. Using a peeler, shave the cheese over the top.

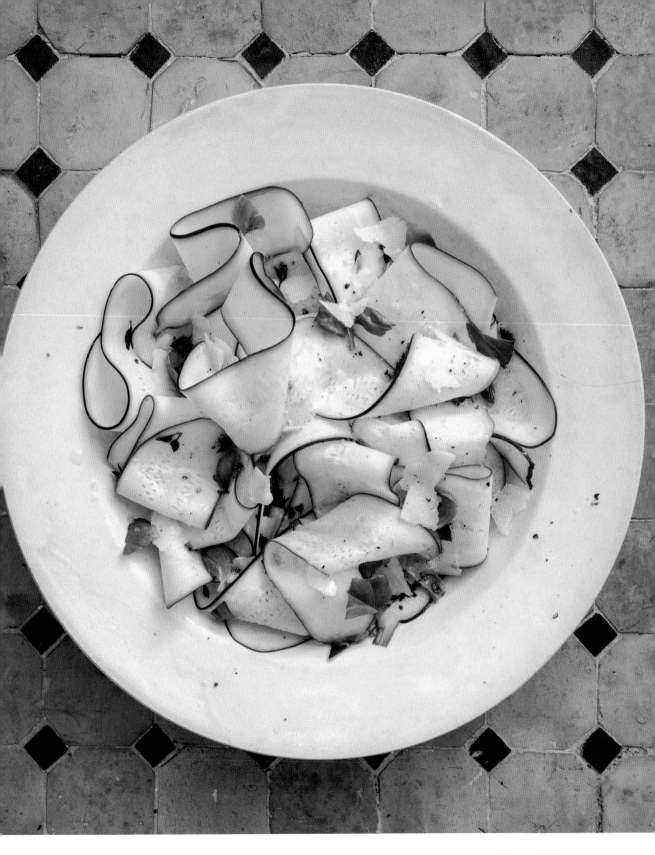

INFO PER SERVING: PROTEIN (G) 4   CARBS (G) 2   SUGAR (G) 2   FAT (G) 8   SATURATED FAT (G) 2   FIBRE (G) 1   SALT (G) 0.1

Makes: **1.5 litres**

 Prep: **10 minutes**

 Cooking time:
about 1 hour

VEGETABLE STOCK

1 tsp olive oil

2 large onions, roughly
chopped

3 large carrots, chopped

200g squash or pumpkin,
unpeeled, diced

4 celery sticks, sliced

2 leeks, sliced

100ml white wine or vermouth

a large thyme sprig

a large parsley sprig

1 bay leaf

a few peppercorns

Stock is a great way of using up any slightly past their best
vegetables you find at the bottom of the fridge – and it will
make your soups and stews taste even better.

Heat the olive oil in a large saucepan. Add all the vegetables and fry them over
a high heat, stirring regularly, until they start to brown and caramelise around the
edges. This will take at least 10 minutes. Add the white wine or vermouth and boil
until it has evaporated away.

Cover the vegetables with 2 litres of water and add the herbs and peppercorns.
Bring to the boil, then turn the heat down to a gentle simmer. Cook the stock,
uncovered, for about an hour, stirring every so often.

Check the stock – the colour should have some depth to it. Strain it through a
colander or a sieve lined with muslin or kitchen paper into a bowl. Store it in the
fridge for up to a week or freeze it.

Makes: **1.5 litres**

Prep: **10 minutes**

Cooking time:
about 3 hours

CHICKEN STOCK

at least 1 chicken carcass,
 pulled apart

4 chicken wings (optional)

1 onion, unpeeled, cut into
 quarters

1 large carrot, cut into large
 chunks

2 celery sticks, roughly
 chopped

1 leek, roughly chopped

1 tsp black peppercorns

3 bay leaves

1 large parsley sprig

1 small thyme sprig

a few garlic cloves, unpeeled
 (optional)

Once you've enjoyed your Sunday roast chicken dinner, don't throw the carcass away. Use it to make a delicious stock to enrich your soups and other dishes. You can also buy chicken carcasses very cheaply at most butchers.

Put the chicken bones and the wings, if using, into a saucepan, just large enough for all the chicken to fit quite snugly. Cover with cold water, bring to the boil, then skim off any foam that collects. Add the remaining ingredients and turn the heat down to a very low simmer. Partially cover the pan with a lid.

Leave the stock to simmer for about 3 hours, then remove the pan from the heat. Strain the stock through a colander or a sieve lined with some muslin or kitchen paper into a bowl.

The stock can be used right away, although it is best to skim off most of the fat that will collect on the top. If you don't need the stock immediately, leave it to cool. The fat will set on top and will be much easier to remove. You can keep the stock in the fridge for up to 5 days or freeze it. If you want to make a larger amount of stock, save up your chicken carcasses in the freezer or add more chicken wings.

INDEX

MASSIVE THANKS

Our brilliant team has helped us produce a book we're so proud of. First off, heartfelt thank yous to the amazing Catherine Phipps, cooking guru extraordinaire, who helps us develop recipes that make all our mouths water. And to our multi-talented photographer Andrew Hayes-Watkins who not only takes great pictures of the food but also makes us look good! Hattie Baker and her assistant Stevie Taylor have both worked their socks off to cook all the food for the photos – huge thanks to them for their skill and hard work. Rachel Vere sourced some beautiful dishes and pans, and Lucie Stericker art-directed the photo shoots and designed the book with her usual style and creative flair. And thanks to Alice Theobald for making us presentable for the photographs.

As always, editor Jinny Johnson has held our hands throughout and made sure everything makes sense. Many thanks, too, to Elise See Tai for proofreading and to Vicki Robinson for compiling the index. Fiona Hunter, expert nutritionist, worked out all the calorie counts and nutritional info for us and we are truly grateful for her input.

Love and thanks also to the Orion team: Vicky Eribo, our wonderful publisher, who has supported us and guided us through the project with enthusiasm and skill, Anna Valentine, Jess Hart, who designed the book cover, Virginia Woolstencroft, Lynsey Sutherland, Helena Fouracre, Jennifer Wilson, Claire Keep and Tierney Witty.

Last but not least, our thanks to the beautiful people at ITG, our management – Nicola Ibison, Roland Carreras and Tasha Hall – and to Barrie Simpson, webmaster, and Iza Orzac, social media star.

What would we do without you? Love you all.

Si and Dave

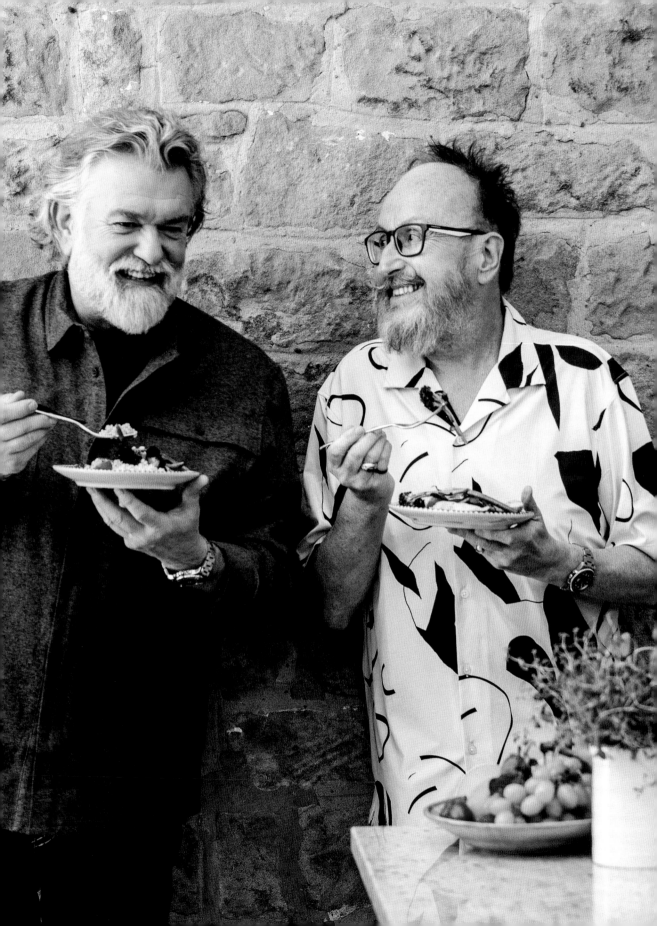

First published in Great Britain in 2024 by Seven Dials,
an imprint of The Orion Publishing Group Ltd
Carmelite House, 50 Victoria Embankment
London EC4Y 0DZ

An Hachette UK Company

10 9 8 7 6 5 4 3 2

A CIP catalogue record for this book is available from the British Library.

ISBN 978 1 3996 0726 0
ISBN (eBook) 978 1 3996 0737 7

Publisher: Vicky Eribo
Recipe consultant: Catherine Phipps
Photography: Andrew Hayes-Watkins
Design and art direction: Lucie Stericker, Studio 7:15
Editor: Jinny Johnson
Food stylist: Hattie Baker
Food stylist's assistant: Stevie Taylor
Prop stylist: Rachel Vere

Groomer: Alice Theobald
Proofreader: Elise See Tai
Indexer: Vicki Robinson
Production manager: Claire Keep
Nutritional consultant: Fiona Hunter, Bsc (Hons)
  Nutrition, Dip Dietetics
Design assistant: Kim McCauley, Studio 7:15

Origination by F1 Colour Ltd, London
Printed in Germany

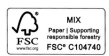

www.orionbooks.co.uk